Creating Effective
Conference Abstracts and Posters
in Biomedicine

Creating Effective Conference Abstracts and Posters in Biomedicine

500 TIPS FOR SUCCESS

JANE FRASER PhD
Independent Scientific Communications Consultant
Jane Fraser Associates Ltd
Altrincham, Cheshire, UK

LOUISE FULLER MA, PhD
Independent Scientific Writer and Writing Skills Trainer
Witney, Oxon, UK

and

GEORGINA HUTBER MA, PhD
Independent Scientific Writer and Writing Skills Trainer
Southampton, Hants, UK

Foreword by
CATHERINE DUNBAR
Manager of the Interactive Education Unit
The Institute of Cancer Research
Sutton, Surrey

Radcliffe Publishing
Oxford • New York

Radcliffe Publishing Ltd
18 Marcham Road
Abingdon
Oxon OX14 1AA
United Kingdom

www.radcliffe-oxford.com
Electronic catalogue and worldwide online ordering facility.

British Library Cataloguing in Publication Data

A catalogue record for this book is available from the British Library.

ISBN-13: 978 184619 311 8

Typeset by Pindar NZ, Auckland, New Zealand
Printed and bound by Hobbs the Printers, Southampton, UK

Contents

Foreword

As a researcher and academic, you need to be able to disseminate and communicate your research work and findings. While many will view writing for peer-reviewed journals as the pinnacle of the academic communication hierarchy, being able to write and present conference abstracts and posters is also extremely important. Taking your work to conferences allows you to meet experts from all around the world, to exchange ideas in person and to network with potential employers and collaborators.

While many of you will have been through the process of submitting a conference abstract and preparing and presenting a poster several or even many times before, there are always ways to improve the process and reduce the level of stress involved! This book is a mine of useful, practical tips covering the entire process – from reading the abstract submission guidelines, through to writing and laying out your poster and creating e-posters. If you are a novice, this is the ideal book to guide you through every step. And even if you consider yourself an expert, there is bound to be some useful information you can glean from the 500 or so tips.

There will be tips you have never considered before that may make the process easier for next time and/or improve the quality of your work. For example, do you know what the protocol is for submitting the same abstract to several conferences? Or when you should and should not use a 'funny' title for your poster? Or how many bullet points you should use in a list on a poster? Or how to ensure your poster is printed as you want it to be? Read on to find the answers to all of these questions and many, many more.

At the Institute of Cancer Research – a specialist research organisation and higher education institution – we pride ourselves on leading the way in training our research students, postdoctoral fellows, scientists and clinicians. Part of this work is ensuring our students and staff have the necessary transferable skills throughout their academic careers and beyond. We are especially keen to promote excellent verbal and written presentation skills (Dr Louise Fuller of Jane Fraser Associates, one of the authors of this book, has run successful courses on writing and publishing skills for the Institute), as it is vital that our scientists can communicate their work with peers, students, funders and the public. Indeed, this is the case for all biomedical researchers and academics. The authors of this book ensure that the practical advice needed to develop these skills is conveyed clearly. Through reading this book, in sequence or by dipping into relevant chapters, you will have all the necessary help with preparing abstracts and posters right at your fingertips.

Catherine Dunbar
Manager of the Interactive Education Unit
The Institute of Cancer Research
Sutton, Surrey
October 2008

Preface

For most biomedical researchers and academics, preparing conference abstracts and posters is an important part of professional life. The fact that you're reading this book suggests that you are already aware of the importance of good conference abstracts and posters in science. You know that your conference abstract can make the difference between acceptance for an oral presentation, a poster presentation – or no presentation at all. You also know that your poster can influence how you – and your research – are perceived by your peers, superiors and potential employers or grant-awarding bodies. This is particularly true at the outset of your career, when you are striving for recognition of your research in an increasingly crowded and competitive arena. So it pays to make sure your conference abstracts and posters are as good as possible.

Abstracts and posters have come a long way since any of the authors were research students – at least in terms of technology. We now have online abstract submission and electronic abstract books, and we have computer programs to help us prepare professional-looking posters with the minimum of effort. Increasingly, posters are presented electronically, as e-posters. We even have digital technology that makes it possible to include video and sound as part of our poster presentations. Much as we may enjoy these tools, we should bear in mind that scientists are sceptical, and a flashy poster cannot conceal dubious data. On the other hand, a well-thought-out abstract or professional-looking poster will help to give your work the best chance of reaching its target audience.

We believe that, with good preparation and practice, all scientists can produce abstracts that act as effective ambassadors for their research. We also believe that a well-designed poster can enhance your professional reputation in addition to communicating your data. This book aims to help you achieve these objectives.

We recognise that scientists have varying needs, so this book is designed for you to use when you are actually preparing a conference abstract or poster. It is intended to answer the most frequent questions and to help you avoid the most common problems and pitfalls. You do not have to read it straight through from beginning to end – just dip into any chapter and you will find a range of tips relevant to the abstract or poster you are preparing right now.

We hope that everyone who reads this book will find useful hints that they can use again and again to help make preparing abstracts and posters easier and reading them more pleasurable. Good luck, and we hope to see your work at future conferences.

For further information on courses on scientific writing and presentation skills, go to www.janefraser.com or contact us at jane@janefraser.com; tel: +44 (0)161 928 6684.

JF, LF and GH
October 2008

About the authors

Dr Jane Fraser, **Dr Louise Fuller** and **Dr Georgina Hutber** work together as Jane Fraser Associates Ltd to provide tailor-made in-house training for publishers, medical communications companies, universities, research institutes and pharmaceutical and biotech companies worldwide. For more information, please visit our website at www.janefraser.com.

Jane started her career as a research scientist but moved into publishing when she realised that she liked writing about the experiments more than she liked doing them! Jane worked as editorial director for two international medical communications agencies, and in the last 20 years she has written, edited and advised on hundreds of abstracts and posters on a variety of scientific topics. Jane founded Jane Fraser Associates in 1991 to offer courses on writing, editing and presentation skills to scientific researchers and publishing professionals. She is also a consulting tutor to the University of Oxford's Continuing Professional Development Centre, where she enjoys helping scientists from many different countries to write abstracts, posters and papers. Jane is the author of three previous books: *Publishing in Biomedicine: 500 tips for success* (Radcliffe Publishing, 1997, revised edition 2008), *Presenting in Biomedicine: 500 tips for success* (Radcliffe Publishing, 2004) and *Professional Proposal Writing* (Ashgate, 1995).

Louise is a scientific writer and trainer with more than 20 years of experience. Louise's degree, PhD and postdoctoral research were carried out at the University of Cambridge. After leaving university life she joined an international medical communications agency. For the last 12 years she has been freelance, working with various medical communications agencies to produce a range of publications, including congress abstracts, posters, slide presentations, clinical and scientific papers, conference reports, press packs, press releases, promotional materials and training manuals. She also mentors and trains professional medical writers and editors working within agencies. Louise now works with Jane Fraser Associates to run workshops and other training sessions on a range of aspects of scientific and medical writing and editing.

After graduating from the University of Oxford, Georgina started her career as a research scientist in biochemistry at the University of Wales, first as a PhD student and then as a postdoctoral fellow. However, she enjoyed writing her PhD thesis and subsequent papers so much that she moved into publishing when the opportunity arose. Georgina worked for several years as an editor, writer, editorial manager and trainer in an international medical communications agency. For the last 18 years she has been working as a freelance medical and scientific editor and writer. She has written clinical and scientific papers, conference reports, abstracts and posters, slide presentations, product monographs, training manuals and press releases. She now makes use of her 25 years' experience of scientific writing and editing in running skills training workshops with Jane Fraser Associates.

Acknowledgements

This book grew out of the questions and suggestions of participants in the courses we have taught on scientific writing, publishing and presenting. Special thanks are therefore due to the Continuing Professional Development Centre and the Department of Medical Sciences at the University of Oxford, the Joint Research Centre Institutes of the European Union, the European Molecular Biology Laboratory, Gothenburg University, the Flanders Institute for Biotechnology, the Royal Veterinary College, the Institute of Cancer Research, the Institute of Genetics and Molecular and Cellular Biology and the Institute for Animal Health.

We are grateful also to many publishers, medical communications agencies and pharmaceutical companies and their staff who have kindly invited us to teach courses. We would also like to mention the numerous mentors, colleagues and clients who helped us to gain our own abstract- and poster-writing skills as professional scientific writers and editors. Thank you all – we continue to learn and hope to keep on adding to our store of tips!

1

Why you need good conference abstracts and posters

For most scientists working in academia or in industry, taking part in scientific conferences is an essential and enjoyable part of professional life. Conferences offer the opportunity to communicate your findings, to exchange ideas, to meet potential new employers – and, in the process, to see new places and have fun! For young scientists especially, writing good conference abstracts and posters is an essential skill that will help to progress your research and promote you and your institution.

A conference abstract is usually a necessity if you want to give a talk or present a poster

For most talks and all posters, you will need to submit an abstract for review by the conference scientific programme committee and have it accepted. So it is worthwhile spending some time making sure that your abstract *will* be accepted. The only talks for which an abstract might not be necessary are very small friendly meetings where everyone attending gives an oral presentation, or major meetings that have some invited 'plenary' talks (review presentations by well-known experts, which do not usually require an abstract). Most of the time, however, the abstract – usually submitted months before the meeting – is an inescapable fact of conference life.

Recognise the importance of your abstract . . .

All too often, abstracts are poorly written or rambling and do not clearly show the conference scientific programme committee that the author has anything interesting to say. By recognising how important the abstract is and spending an adequate amount of time planning and writing it, you will be able to avoid this pitfall.

. . . And the need to present your data well

Selection committees look for good science. If the abstract is confusing or incomplete, the standard of the research may be underestimated. A well-written abstract allows the scientific quality of a study to be assessed objectively.

Your abstract may be used to decide whether you give a talk or a poster . . .

Some conferences have a policy of accepting all abstracts submitted but use the abstracts to decide which contributions should be presented orally and which as posters. In general, the better the abstract, the better your chances of being asked to give an oral presentation.

. . . Or whether you get any sort of presentation at all

Other meetings are highly competitive and reject some abstracts altogether. That could mean not only that your work is not communicated, but also that you do not get to go to the meeting.

'No acceptance' may mean 'no attendance'

From the organiser's point of view, it is usually perfectly acceptable for delegates to attend a conference without giving a talk or showing a poster, as long as the registration fee is paid. However, in practice, many institutions or grant-awarding bodies only cover the costs of attendance if you are giving a talk or presenting a poster.

Some conferences print every abstract submitted in an abstract book or on CD-ROM

A few conferences print all abstracts submitted in an abstract book or include them on a CD-ROM or web page, even if the authors are not offered a talk or poster.

This may help individuals to get funding to attend the meeting, even if they are not presenting their data.

A good abstract stimulates interest in your oral presentation or poster

During the conference, abstracts are usually available to all participants via a printed abstract book, in electronic format, or both. Participants can search the abstracts to decide which talks they want to attend and which posters they want to visit. A clearly written abstract encourages people to come to your talk or look at your poster and to discuss your work with you.

In competitive fields, an abstract or poster helps to establish the originality of an idea

No one can actually 'own' an idea in science. However (rightly or wrongly), scientists attach importance to originality – you get respect from being the first group to publish something new and exciting. As it often takes a long time to progress from doing the research to having a paper published, it sometimes helps to 'stake a claim' through an abstract, especially if the abstract is available in the public domain after the meeting. The abstract is only a small first step, however; for your work to be taken seriously by the scientific community, you must go on to publish the full paper in a peer-reviewed journal.

Conference abstracts may help to publicise research even after the meeting is over

Conference abstracts that remain on websites after the meeting is over may help alert online searchers to your research. Some conferences (especially society meetings) publish their abstracts in a supplement to a learned journal, and these abstracts may be retrieved through databases such as PubMed.

Conference abstracts can sometimes be cited in papers

Published abstracts may be cited in other people's papers even if the full paper has not been published yet. However, some journals only allow citations to recent conference abstracts, because it is expected that if the work is good enough to survive peer review it will have been published in a journal within a year or two of the conference abstract first appearing.

A poster presentation is definitely better than no presentation

Some people feel disappointed if they are offered 'only' a poster presentation rather than a talk. There is no need to be downhearted if this happens to you – poster presentations offer a useful means of communicating your work and getting to a scientific meeting to hear new data and make new contacts, including potential research collaborators and employers. Posters can sometimes even offer advantages over an oral presentation (*see* below).

Sometimes a poster is preferable to a talk

Some conferences give you the chance to state whether you prefer to give a talk or present a poster. There might be times when you would rather give a poster than a talk. This might be because:

- you don't like giving talks (better to get over this if you can; giving talks is an inescapable fact of academic life)
- your methods or results are very complex, and the time allowed for talks is too short to give a meaningful explanation (be sure that this is really the case)
- you feel that your work is too preliminary to present orally, but you would welcome the opportunity to present it as a poster and receive comments and advice
- you want to use a poster as a means of attracting constructive criticism on the design of a study protocol
- you want to raise awareness of the existence of an ongoing study even before you have any results
- you want to invite people to participate in a collaborative venture such as a multicentre trial or a disease registry that is better explained in a poster.

Posters create opportunities to meet people and discuss your work

A poster presentation may be your first chance of getting your work into the public domain. This applies whether it consists of data, ideas or just the existence of your ongoing study, even if you do not yet have many results. It will give you the opportunity to discuss your work with other scientists, and you may gain new insights and new interpretations that will help with ongoing work. However, try not be disappointed if readers do not stop to talk – a well-prepared poster will still have given them useful information and something to think about.

A poster promotes you and your institution

If you are offered a poster presentation at a scientific meeting, this is useful material for your curriculum vitae or for grant applications. Just being at the conference is useful promotion for you and your institution or company. So remember to make it clear on your poster who you are and where you work.

A well-designed poster will attract people in a busy conference hall

A poster is very different from a paper for publication. It has to capture attention across a crowded hall and encourage readers to come close enough to read it. And once the reader has arrived, the poster has to tell its story simply and quickly, as readers are busy and will have many other posters to visit. They do not want to spend much time deciphering the message. So for you, time spent in designing a good poster is time well spent.

A poor poster is worse than no poster at all

It is worth remembering that a poorly produced poster could have a negative effect on perceptions of you or your institution. Take time to plan *both* the content and the layout/design of your poster. Ask your friends and colleagues what they think about your ideas and for suggestions on how you could improve it – before it is too late!

2

Your abstract: first steps

Before you start to write your abstract, it is important to check out any relevant rules and regulations and to make some important decisions regarding matters such as authorship and selection of data.

Before you start, think about authorship

If you are writing an abstract for a conference, it is probable that you have been closely involved in much of the research and feel that you have a major investment in getting it published. However, it is likely that you did not work alone. Anyone who contributed substantively to the research you want to present should be an author on the abstract.

Decide who will be the presenting author . . .

The presenting author must be the person who will attend the conference and give the oral or poster presentation. Will that be you? Check that you are free for the dates of the conference. If not, either change conference or change presenting author. In general, conferences disapprove of changes to the presenting author after abstract submission.

. . . And agree on the order of other authors

The presenting author is usually the first author on the abstract. Ideally, other authors should be listed according to their level of contribution to the study. For some studies this will be obvious, but sometimes (in collaborative studies, for example) there can be differences of opinion. Discuss the order of authorship with your co-authors as early as possible to avoid any subsequent disagreements.

Be aware of why abstracts are accepted . . .

The most important factors for abstract acceptance for a prestigious and competitive meeting are the quality, novelty, reliability and clinical and scientific importance of your work. So if you have conducted well-designed scientific or clinical investigations, you are three parts of the way to acceptance.

. . . And rejected

However, even the best work may be presented badly. Apart from not conforming to specific submission instructions, abstracts may be rejected because they are written in a disorganised manner or they contain old information or a vague discussion of the importance of the topic area.

Write the abstract so as to maximise your chances of acceptance

Rightly or wrongly, reviewers may be inclined to look more favourably on abstracts that are well structured and written in good English. In the worst cases, serious errors in language can make the science hard to understand. If English is not your native language, it may be worthwhile showing your draft to someone who can edit it for spelling, grammar and style.

Select your conference carefully

Each scientific conference has its own scientific focus and set of objectives. For example, some will be largely clinically focused and others will focus primarily on cellular research. Some will see themselves as having an educational focus and others as being at the cutting edge of research. To maximise your chances of acceptance, pick an appropriate conference for your data. If you are not sure, ask your colleagues and look on the conference website.

Discuss the most appropriate session with your co-authors

Even at the same conference, some topic sessions may be more competitive than others. If your data are not very exciting, it might be better to submit your abstract for a less popular topic into which it still fits. You may want to discuss the most appropriate session with your co-authors – if so, do this as early as possible, just in case there is disagreement and you need time to finalise the decision.

Get a copy of the submission instructions . . .

The instructions for preparation and submission of abstracts are usually available on the conference website. Failure to follow the rules could result in your abstract being immediately returned to you for amendment, wasting both your time and the scientific committee's time. Your abstract could even be rejected completely. Nowadays, abstracts are usually submitted electronically via the conference website. This ensures that all abstracts can be published in a standard format.

. . . And follow them carefully

Read the instructions carefully, noting whether a word count or character count is specified and whether you are allowed figures and tables in the abstract. The instructions may tell you whether the abstract has to be structured (i.e. with section headings), whether authors' names and affiliations are considered part of your character or word count, whether you have to follow a particular format for names and affiliations and whether you have to include your email address.

Check whether a submission fee is required . . .

A small number of conferences may charge an abstract submission fee. This helps to cover the costs of the meeting and may help to ensure that everyone who submits an abstract to a highly competitive meeting is serious about presenting at the conference. However, at present, submission payments are the exception rather than the rule.

. . . And make sure you have funding for this

Fees are normally small, but if you don't have much grant left you may want to submit to an alternative conference. It is a good idea to add a small amount for submission fees into any grant application to cover this eventuality.

If you need a scientific sponsor for your abstract, act quickly

Some conferences require a member of the learned society that runs the conference to sponsor each abstract submission. There is often a limit on the number of abstracts that one person can sponsor, so act quickly to sign up your sponsor.

Submit the abstract on time

It pays to make sure that you know when the submission deadline is. Deadlines are often ruthlessly imposed, and late abstracts may be rejected irrespective of their scientific merit.

Note that deadlines may be more lenient for hotline sessions

Some conferences may arrange hotline or late-breaking sessions for very important studies if it is known for certain that results will be available by the date of the meeting. The submission deadline for such a session will be later than for the bulk of the abstracts. However, unless you are certain that your study will be considered sufficiently important for a hotline session, it would be unwise to count on your abstract being accepted at the later deadline. Talk to the conference scientific programme committee if you are likely to have important late-breaking data – they will let you know if the data are going to be suitable for late-breaker status.

Decide what to do if you do not have any results yet

Conference abstracts often have to be submitted many months before the actual conference, when scientific investigations are still continuing. It used to be common to see conference abstracts in the 'indicative' format. This format tells you what question the study was designed to answer and something about the methods but gives no results. You will probably have seen abstracts that start or conclude with 'Results will be presented for . . .'. However, many scientific programme committees, particularly for very competitive conferences, now refuse to accept indicative abstracts in order to avoid last-minute withdrawals for lack of results. If you want to submit an indicative abstract, it is advisable to check the committee's policy.

Check whether you can give interim results

If your work is still in progress, you may have baseline data or preliminary results that you could present in an abstract. For example, the scientific programme committee may be willing to accept an analysis of data from a smaller number of patients than the complete study or of just some of the parameters you measured. If the committee can be convinced that you will be able to present the full results at the meeting, they may be satisfied. Again, however, it may be advisable to check the policy before submitting your abstract.

Consider submitting an abstract to more than one conference

Contrary to what many people think, it is usually quite acceptable to present the same research at more than one conference. Different audiences will give you different kinds of feedback. However, it is a good idea to pitch the content of each abstract in a slightly different way to match the focus of each conference. Don't forget to alter the title to reflect the changes you have made. Check with the conference 'Instructions to authors', however – for some sessions it is required that your work is being presented in public for the first time.

3

Your abstract: planning, structure and title

Before you start writing your abstract, you need to plan it carefully. Because it is a short piece of writing, it can be tricky to fit everything in, and you need to maximise the impact of each element. The title is particularly important because it is the first thing that the scientific committee and the conference participants read.

Plan before you write

Before you start writing, ask yourself the four 'Whats' about your work.

- What was the purpose of this study?
- What did I do?
- What did I find, identify or learn?
- What is the importance of my findings?

This approach will also help when you come to preparing your oral or poster presentation.

Include all the key components of your study

Your abstract should contain all the key components of your work. For experimental work, you typically need:

- title
- background/objective

- methods
- results
- conclusions.

Consider a structured abstract

A structured abstract is one that is written under a number of standard headings, which reflect the key components of the work. This makes it more informative for the reader and also facilitates writing. Many submission instructions for conference abstracts recommend using a structured abstract, though it may not be compulsory. Even if you do not actually put the headings in the final abstract, using them in your draft can help you to focus your thoughts and start writing. An example of a structured abstract is given in Appendix 1.

Follow the CONSORT guidelines if you are reporting a clinical trial

For reporting randomised controlled clinical trials, some conferences now follow the CONSORT guidelines (www.consort-statement.org). You may therefore be required to include extra details, such as the funding source and trial registration number, in addition to specific information about the background/objective, methods, results and conclusions. Like journals, conference organisers may tell you to use a specific structure for your abstract, so check their instructions carefully.

Make your title as informative as possible . . .

The title is the first thing that reviewers and conference participants read, so writing a good title will not only help to get your abstract noticed when you submit it, it may also persuade people to come to your presentation. A good title is clear, informative and includes the key components of your work, such as patient group/animals/cells/genes, disease, experimental approach, dependent and independent variables and outcomes. For example, *'The effect of X on Y in patients with P: a double-blind, randomised, controlled trial'*.

. . . And the right length

Very short or very long titles are not recommended (and a very long title may use up valuable words from the total allowed). It is easier to write the title after you have written the abstract, and you will then also know how much space you have left. There are often character limits on titles of abstracts. This is not a challenge to reach the limit; it is fine to have fewer characters than this.

When drafting your abstract title, consider your poster

When you are drafting the title of your abstract, bear in mind that the same title will be used on your poster (*see* Chapter 11). So you need to think about the number of words you use, and how a long or a short abstract title will appear on a poster.

Make the title simple and straightforward . . .

Do not be afraid that simple, clear language will appear 'unscientific'. You do not have to use complex language just because you are dealing with complex science. Try writing your title several different ways until you feel it is clear. Delete any unnecessary words, such as '*Studies on . . .*' or '*An analysis of . . .*'.

. . . But make it scientifically interesting

To create interest in your abstract, the title should either state the findings of your study (a declarative title, *see* below) or should hint at them. It is fine to be controversial, as long as your data are also controversial. Think about the final title – if you were a delegate at the meeting, would this title draw you to this poster?

Consider using a declarative title

A declarative title is one that states the key result of the study, for example, '*Vitalimix increases exercise capacity in gerbils*'. If you already have a clear, convincing conclusion when you are writing the abstract, a declarative title can be helpful to the reader and can be a useful way of saving words (as a declarative title is often shorter than a non-declarative title). However, not all scientific programme committees accept declarative titles, so you should check the submission guidelines.

Be very thoughtful before you choose a 'funny' title

It might be tempting to choose an amusing title in the hope of attracting people to your presentation or poster. However, such titles are seldom appropriate nowadays, for several reasons.

- Busy conference abstract review committees and conference attendees are likely to be annoyed by titles that do not allow them to see immediately what the study was about.
- Jokes or puns may be misunderstood by people who are not native speakers of the language concerned (usually English).
- A 'funny' title may not contain the search terms that will allow people to find your talk or poster through electronic programme searches.

- If a company has sponsored your research, they may not want you to be too light-hearted. They have taken you, and the subject of your research, seriously enough to give you money.

It's best to keep 'funny' titles for informal talks within your own institution or for student posters where no abstract is needed and there's no selection committee to consider.

Put the most important words near the beginning of your title

For maximum impact, try to make the first few words of your title the ones that will attract readers interested in your subject. Sometimes you may be able to use a colon or a dash in the middle of the title in order to get the words in the right order. For example, *'Grottomycin versus scabicillin in acute sinusitis in elderly patients: a randomised controlled trial'* is more attention-grabbing than *'A randomised controlled trial of . . .'*.

If necessary, you can use well-known abbreviations or acronyms in your title to save space . . .

It is usually acceptable in conference abstracts (even in titles) to use common abbreviations such as DNA or HIV without spelling them out on first use, provided you are sure that your readers will understand them. In fact, conference abstracts often use common abbreviations in the title to save space.

. . . But spell out uncommon abbreviations

Always spell out uncommon abbreviations on first use. Normally, you would then give the abbreviation in brackets immediately after the words. If abbreviations are explained in this way in the title, you don't have to explain them again in the text. If people are not familiar with the abbreviated version of a term, failure to spell it out in the title might lead to your abstract being missed if the conference abstract book is searchable online.

Use acronyms sensibly

Pivotal clinical studies often use acronyms (e.g. HOPE, MOTIV) rather than writing out a lengthy trial description. If your data are part of a major and very well-known study, you can use the acronym without spelling it out in full. However, if the study is new, you must spell out the acronym the first time that it is used. Do not create an acronym simply to save space in your abstract.

Include key words in the title

If you want conference participants to come to your presentation, you should include key words in the title that will attract them. For example, *'Effects of Necrotiplan and Vitalimix on exercise capacity in gerbils'* would be better than something vague such as *'Effects of dietary supplements on exercise capacity in rodents'*. Key words in the title may also be used to compile the index to the abstract book and as search terms on the conference website or in online databases.

Test your title on your colleagues

Once you are happy with your title, try it out on some colleagues – do they agree that it is clear and simple?

Use the 3-second rule

Anyone reading your abstract should be able to read and understand your title within 3 seconds. Try this out on yourself and your colleagues. If it takes longer than 3 seconds, redraft the title.

4

Writing your abstract

An abstract submitted to a scientific meeting should be a brief but comprehensive summary of the presentation you intend to make, whether oral or poster. Once you have written your abstract, use the checklist in Appendix 2 to make sure that you are on the right track.

Keep the background section short

Writers too often write several introductory sentences that are vague and general. The conference participants are presumably all interested in the overall topic area, so the background needs to be targeted to their likely level of knowledge. Quite often, a single sentence will be sufficient, though you can expand it if you are short of data to put in the abstract!

State the objective clearly

A single sentence should be enough to tell the reader what you were trying to find out, i.e. your research question or hypothesis. You may be able to include some of the method used in this sentence, for example, '*A randomised, double-blind, placebo-controlled study was conducted to determine . . .*'. You do not then need to repeat this information in the methods section. It is important that the objective does not just repeat or paraphrase the title – that is a waste of your word allocation because it does not provide the reader with additional specific information about what you were trying to find out.

Reconsider if you have more than one objective

It is probably best to just focus on one objective in your abstract, otherwise you may find it difficult not only to write a good abstract in the allotted space, but also to present the data well at the conference. If you find you have more than one objective, reconsider your abstract and potential presentation. It may be possible to submit more than one abstract describing different aspects of your work.

Unless you developed or evaluated a new method, keep the methods section brief . . .

Unless the whole point of your presentation is to describe a new method or to evaluate an existing method, you should keep the details of your methods to the minimum necessary to understand the results. However, if you only have preliminary data to report, you may need to expand the methods to fill the space!

. . . But make sure you include all the relevant details

If you do not supply enough detail about your methods, the abstract reviewers and conference participants will not be able to judge whether your results are valid. They have no other material on which to base their judgement (unlike a published paper, which provides more detail in the body of the text). You should describe the genes, antibodies, cells/organisms or patients studied; the study design (if you have not already put this in the objective); the doses of drugs and their length of administration; brief details of any assays or laboratory tests used; and the main outcome measures of clinical studies.

You can usually leave out the statistical methods, unless the main focus is on statistics

The statistical methods can often be omitted from an abstract, provided they are standard. For example, if you present hazard ratios or mean differences, it is not necessary to explain that you used proportional hazards models or linear regression. If you have used modified statistical methods, you should state them briefly.

Think about what you would want to know about the methods

It is always a good idea to think about what you would ask if you were reading someone else's conference abstract. Use this as a guide to what to include in the methods section.

Every result should have a corresponding method

Every set of data in the results must also be represented in the methods section and vice versa. The overall flow of your abstract will be compromised if you include results out of context.

Present your results clearly . . .

Your results are the most important part of the abstract, so it is important that you state them clearly. You should avoid long and confusing sentences and follow a logical order. For example, in a clinical study, you could start with describing the study participants by giving actual numbers for demographic data, then give the results for the primary outcome measure followed by the secondary outcome measures (if you have space).

. . . And precisely

It is very important that you present your results precisely so that the abstract reviewers (and conference participants, if you get to that stage) can assess the quality of your findings. It is not very informative to say 'Asthma was highly prevalent in these children' if you do not give numbers to back up your statement. One of the most common failings of abstracts is lack of numerical data. Glossing over a lack of results by making vague statements will not help your abstract to be accepted.

. . . And accurately

If you state in the methods that you have adjusted the variables you measured for confounding factors in a multivariate analysis, you should give only the adjusted estimates in the results, not the crude estimates.

. . . And focus on those results that relate to the study objective

You do not have to report all your results in the abstract. There is a temptation to put in all the results that are significant. However, it is more important that you show that you have addressed the study objective and that you report the outcomes that you considered important before the analysis, even if your findings are not significant.

In clinical studies, do not forget any important adverse events

You may not have been specifically looking for adverse events, and/or your study may not have been adequately powered to evaluate their incidence statistically. But if any important adverse events of an intervention occurred, you should mention them.

Think about how to deal with negative results

You may not have been able to show what you wanted but still feel that your negative results are important and worth presenting. However, it is generally more difficult to get negative results accepted than positive ones, so it would be better to present mainly positive data with just a few negative data if you can. If your main results are negative, you should be able to explain in just one or two sentences why they are important and/or the reasons for their being negative.

If allowed, consider using a figure or table to present your results

Electronic submission of abstracts often means that you can include a figure or table in your abstract. The submission guidelines on the conference website should tell you if you can include a figure or table and, if so, how to insert it. Only use a figure or table if it improves the presentation of your data – ask yourself whether, as a reader, you would find it quicker to interpret the table or figure or to read text. If you do include a figure or table, select the data carefully to deliver the key message or summarise the most important findings. Put all other details in the text.

Give sample sizes as well as percentages

To help the reader to make an informed judgement of the validity of your data, you need to provide the sample size as well as the percentage, for example, '*3/30 patients (10%)*'. You can give the sample size only once, if it does not vary, but if it does vary, make this clear when you give the relevant data.

Give actual data as well as p values

It is not sufficient just to say '*Significantly more gerbils in the Vitalimix group than in the Necrotiplan group could run 1 km (p<0.05)*'. You need to give the actual data as well: '*Significantly more gerbils in the Vitalimix group than in the Necrotiplan group could run 1 km (86% vs 56%; p<0.05)*'. Confidence intervals may be more useful than p values, so give them plus the p value if you have space. If you are short of space, give the confidence intervals in preference.

Be accurate and consistent with units

Use SI units wherever relevant. Be consistent; if you begin talking about measuring something in mg, do not switch to g or μg later on. If you are stating a dosage of a drug or chemical, always give both the units of the individual dose and the regimen or timing of administration.

SI abbreviations never need to be spelled out

SI abbreviations such as mg (milligram) or L (litre) never need to be spelled out, wherever in the abstract they occur.

Use your common sense for other abbreviations

You have more freedom to use abbreviations in the main text of a conference abstract than you do in a journal abstract. Unless the scientific programme committee says otherwise, you can use common abbreviations, e.g. DNA or PCR, without spelling them out first time. If you coin an abbreviation to save space in the abstract, spell it out on first use, and make sure that it can be intuitively recognised and not confused with standard abbreviations. Always spare a thought for your readers; overuse of abbreviations can make an abstract difficult to read. Don't *you* just hate the kind of conference abstract that says '*PDQ was used to compare the OP of ABC and XYZ at D3 in HB*'?

Use the word 'significance' with care

In general, readers will assume that 'significant' refers to statistics, so you can save space by saying *significant difference* or *significantly different*, rather than *statistically significant difference*. But equally, you should avoid using terms like *clinical significance*, as this may cause confusion. You can usually find another word to express your meaning, such as *clinical importance* or *clinically relevant*.

Present a clear conclusion

It helps the reader to know the 'bottom line', if there is one, so if you have a conclusion, you should state it clearly. '*This study shows that Vitalimix is better than Necrotiplan at maintaining the health of gerbils. It is therefore a valuable addition to standard gerbil food.*' You should try to avoid simply repeating data, as that wastes space and adds nothing to your abstract.

State any *important* implications (optional) . . .

If your findings are really likely to change clinical practice or to change the way scientists view the topic, there is no reason why you should not say so in the abstract. Otherwise, there is no need to say anything. You should definitely avoid statements like '*More research is needed*' – it always is – or '*This study has important implications for gerbil welfare*'.

. . . But avoid lengthy discussion

Other than a brief, optional statement of any important implications of your work, you do not normally need a discussion in a conference abstract. You wouldn't normally expect to start talking about how your work compares with others' studies, for example. However, you might have some brief discussion in abstracts about theoretical studies or studies from which no simple conclusions can be drawn. You might also need a short discussion if your study shows something so different from preceding research that some explanation of possible reasons is clearly needed.

Be sure to 'sell' your study . . .

You may be able to increase your chance of acceptance by submitting an abstract that makes it clear why the research question is important/interesting/original.

. . . But don't overstate your case

Although you should highlight the originality of your work, you should not (at least at this stage) make it sound as though it might win the Nobel Prize. Although you can mention important implications for science or clinical medicine, you should only do so if your results justify it. Even pioneer breakthrough studies require independent confirmation, and if your results really are outstanding, they will speak for themselves.

Use appropriate tenses

It is conventional to use the present tense for established facts (as in the background section) and for generalisations (such as your conclusions). However, the past tense is used for specific actions and findings by the authors (i.e. methods and results). Your objectives sentence may even contain both past and present tenses! You will be familiar with this convention from your reading, even if you have never thought about it before. So you might write: 'Chocolate consumption is (*present, generalisation*) known to affect mood in research students. To determine whether this effect depends (*present, seeking to make a generalisation*) on the presence of cocoa solids in chocolate, we compared (*past, method*) the effects on mood of dark chocolate (70% cocoa solids) with those of white chocolate (0% cocoa solids). The Happiness Rating Scale was used (*past, method*). No difference was found (*past, result*) between the two types of chocolate. We conclude (*present, generalisation*) that cocoa solids do not contribute (*present, conclusion*) to the effect of chocolate on mood in research students.'

Use references if you really want to

Most journals have an absolute rule against citing references in an abstract. In a conference abstract, however, there is no reason why you should not include one or two key references if you feel that it is worthwhile. Otherwise they just take up valuable word space. If you do use references, keep them short by including only the first author (use *et al.* for others) and omitting the title of the paper.

Finally, edit your abstract thoroughly to make it fit . . .

When you have included all of the above elements, you will almost certainly find that your abstract is too long. Usually all that is required is a thorough edit to eliminate waste words. Look first at your background section – it is often possible to simply delete the entire first sentence. After that, edit the remainder of the abstract according to the rules of clear, concise writing to reduce the number of words without losing the meaning.

- Use short sentences.
- Use short, simple words.
- Avoid technical jargon.
- Be very specific in your choice of words.
- Use the active voice wherever possible ('*Aspirin reduced inflammation*' rather than '*Inflammation was reduced by aspirin*').
- Do not be afraid to use '*we measured*' rather than '*a measurement was performed*'.

. . . And make sure it is self-contained

The abstract review committee and the conference participants only know what you tell them, so make sure that after editing is complete, your abstract still tells the whole story. Make sure that you have defined all the abbreviations that need to be defined and that you have not included methods for which you give no results or vice versa.

Ask a colleague with an eye for detail to read it . . .

You and your co-authors will have worked hard on the study and on drafting the abstract. However, it is possible to become so close to the data that you become blind to obvious errors of scientific thought or use of language. Ask a colleague with knowledge of your field – but not in-depth knowledge of your data – to read your abstract.

. . . And give clear instructions for critiquing the abstract

Ask your colleague to read the abstract as critically as possible. Instruct them to look for problems and errors in:

- the logic of the abstract
- the balance of the different sections
- the link between the objectives and the conclusions
- the presentation of the data
- readability
- 'understandability'
- spelling and grammar.

. . . And accept the criticisms and take action

If your abstract comes back covered in suggestions, do not take offence; use this as a learning exercise and adapt your abstract accordingly. If you make many changes, you should let someone else read the abstract before deciding that you have a final version. The chances are that you will have introduced at least one spelling error while redrafting the abstract.

Make sure that your co-authors read the abstract before submission

Each of your co-authors must be willing to take responsibility for the data and conclusions contained in the abstract. It is essential that all authors have read and are happy with the content.

Reread the final version of your abstract

Are you happy with it? Have the changes from co-authors and colleagues improved it? Does it strike you as an interesting, well-conducted and worthwhile study? If you were a member of the conference scientific programme committee, would you accept it? If you can answer 'yes' to all these questions, the next step is submission to the conference of your choice.

5

Submitting your abstract

In addition to writing a great abstract (*see* Chapter 4), you need to submit it effectively. Nowadays this is usually done online. This chapter offers some tips on online submission and discusses what happens once your abstract is accepted – or rejected.

Familiarise yourself with the submission process

Submission sites usually allow you to create an online draft that will not be submitted to the conference until you press the 'submit' button. You can access the draft abstract as many times as you like and make as many changes as you like, but no further changes are possible once you have pressed 'submit'. Smaller conferences often accept abstracts as attachments to email.

Set up an online account as soon as possible . . .

To take a look at the submission process, you will usually have to set up an online account. Even if you have not written the abstract yet, it is a good idea to do this early. This is especially important if this is your first submission to a particular meeting – you do not want to discover on the day of the deadline that you are missing a critical piece of information.

. . . And do not forget your username and password

It is very annoying to know that you have entered data into a draft submission and then not to be able to access that information when you come to edit or submit the abstract. Conference submission sites often do not supply forgotten usernames and passwords, so write them down somewhere safe!

Check all required elements of the submission

Read every page of the submission website – even if you have to enter dummy information to move through the pages. The submission requirements for every conference are slightly different, and it is often author details that differ most. Some conferences require specific information, such as authors' scientific/medical degrees, dates of birth, full postal addresses, email addresses and financial disclosures or other potential conflicts of interest, whereas others do not.

If you need information or agreement from co-authors or sponsors, give them time to provide it

If you need information from colleagues, get this as soon as possible. You do not want lack of a simple detail to hold up your submission.

Check how your abstract will be assessed

Sometimes you may be asked to submit the authors' names and affiliations in a separate file to ensure that your abstract is assessed in a 'blind' manner by the reviewing committee.

Make sure you know how to upload author details, text, figures and tables

For abstracts themselves, it is usually possible to 'cut and paste' text directly from a word-processing package. Some conferences require that a table or graph is uploaded as an image file, such as a .tif or a .jpg, but others have data-management systems that require you to re-create your table online. You will usually have to type in the details for each author and highlight who is the presenting author.

Consider how to present equations

It is usually a good idea to upload equations as an image file, as most online systems will not be able to handle the formatting requirements of an equation.

Proofread your abstract before pressing 'submit' . . .

Make sure that you carefully proofread your entire abstract, including the title, the author names, the author affiliations and the body text. Some submission sites allow you to print out a page for proofreading. If so, do a word-for-word check against a paper copy of your original manuscript. Sometimes you will have to proofread from a paper copy to an onscreen version. If you have to do this, go as slowly as possible, as it is harder to spot errors.

Remove any dummy copy

If you have entered dummy information into the abstract submission site, it is all too easy to leave it there and then to have strange information appearing in the final abstract. Make sure that you keep track of what information you have added and check that the final versions of the title, author names and affiliations, abstract body text, choice of session and any transparency declarations are the actual submission versions.

Check for missing words and numbers

It is easy to make 'cut and paste' errors when putting your abstract onto the conference website. Check that every word is present and that you have not duplicated any text accidentally.

Check data in tables

This is particularly important if you have had to input a table using data-management software. It is very easy to mistype numbers in tables or to omit column or row headings.

Look for errors in formatting

Many abstract submission sites have only limited flexibility for formatting. Some cannot handle even standard formatting, such as bold, italics, subscripts or super-scripts. Many cannot read special symbols, such as Greek letters or letters with accents. Look for any strange spacing in your text. A special symbol may have been lost. If your data are in $\mu g/mL$, you may want to change the units to mg/L to avoid potential formatting errors.

Read the online instructions for specifying formatting

Some sites tell you how to specify a particular piece of formatting. For example, m² could be m<2>. Although this looks odd, make sure you follow the online rules so that your abstract is consistent with all the others.

If you edit online, check the word count before submitting

It is very tempting to try to perfect your abstract online, particularly if you have late input from colleagues. Beware! Many online systems will simply truncate your abstract if it is too long. It is your responsibility to ensure that your abstract is the correct length. Truncated abstracts will usually not be considered by the scientific programme committee.

Choose the right session

For many conferences you will be asked to indicate in which topic area your abstract belongs. This helps the scientific programme committee to group submissions and to ensure a balance of material presented during the conference. Online systems normally provide a drop-down menu from which you can choose your session.

Do not leave submission until the last minute

Conference websites often have high traffic levels in the few days before the submission deadline. This can mean that the website responds more slowly, which can be frustrating and time-consuming for you. There have been instances of conference web servers crashing on the deadline day due to over-demand. This could leave you wondering if your submission really made it, or worse, having to resubmit even closer to the deadline.

Check your email for an acknowledgement . . .

Most systems automatically send an email to acknowledge online submission. If you do not receive an email within 24 hours, check the online submission system. Contact the conference organisers as soon as possible if you are at all unsure whether your abstract has been submitted successfully.

. . . And for an acceptance

Keep a note of when you should receive an email to tell you whether your abstract has been accepted for an oral presentation or poster so that you can check up if necessary.

Keep a note of which abstracts have been accepted

If you belong to a very prolific research group that submits numerous abstracts to different conferences, it's easy to lose track of which abstracts have been accepted and which are still under consideration. Have some way of keeping track so that you don't have to go looking among your old emails to find out where you stand with your various submissions.

You may be able to withdraw and resubmit before the deadline if urgent changes are needed

After submission, you cannot usually make corrections to the abstract. However, if you really need to change the abstract (because the speaker details have changed or you have found an error, for example), you may be able to withdraw it and submit a new corrected version. This only applies before the submission deadline is reached. After the deadline, it may be possible to withdraw the abstract but not to replace it.

If your abstract is rejected, submit it to another conference

An abstract may be rejected for many reasons, not all of which mean that the data or indeed the abstract were poor (though you should reflect on your data and writing style before progressing). It could simply be that there were too many submissions for that conference. Alternatively, it is possible that you chose the conference because it was at the right time for your schedule (or in a really nice place!) and your data were not an obvious fit with the aims of the scientific programme committee. Do not get downhearted by a rejection – simply submit your data to another suitable meeting.

Rework your abstract to suit the needs of a new conference

When you submit your abstract to a new conference, do not simply send in the same text – make sure that you read the submission instructions for the new meeting and edit your abstract accordingly. If you leave the formatting instructions for one meeting in the text for another, the second scientific programme committee will know that you have had the abstract rejected previously and might look more critically at your data.

Do not forget to register

Conferences usually specify that to present a talk or poster you must be registered for the meeting. Sometimes you are required to register and pay your attendance fee before submitting an abstract. If this is not the case, remember that acceptance of your abstract does not mean that you are automatically registered for the meeting. If you are not sure that you will want or be able to go to the meeting unless your abstract is accepted, you may be able to leave registering until your abstract is accepted. But don't leave it too late – a conference may be fully subscribed before the closing date for registration.

6

Your poster: first steps

Well done – you have already cleared the first hurdle by getting your abstract accepted at a conference and being allocated a slot at a poster session. Now the task ahead is to write and produce the poster and get it safely to the meeting. This section gives you some tips on things to think about before you start putting pen to paper or fingers to keyboard.

Before you start, read the guidelines
Every conference publishes guidelines for poster production. Some meetings provide excellent detailed instructions, but others do not. If you are unclear about anything, telephone or email the organisers. Never start to write or produce a poster unless you fully understand the conference guidelines.

Check the language of the conference
Make sure that you write the poster in the correct language. If it is not your first language, work closely with a colleague or friend to ensure that your poster is well written. The person who edits the poster should have the language of the conference as their first language.

Check the size of the poster board

You should print your poster so that it is smaller than the poster board – try not to have sections of the poster hanging off the bottom of the board. If you are unsure about sizing, talk to the conference organisers. Some instructions will indicate the maximum usable area of the poster board.

- You are not obliged to fill all the area available on the poster board.
- In the US, poster boards are often 4 ft × 8 ft (1.2 m × 2.4 m).
- The most common poster size is A0 (84 cm × 119 cm).

Check whether your poster is supposed to be in landscape or portrait format

For some reason, landscape format seems to be the most popular at clinical conferences, whereas portrait format seems more popular in basic sciences. However, you should always check. The wrong format can look silly on the poster board. You don't want it to be overlapping the edges of the board at the sides or flapping feebly at the bottom.

Build a mental picture of the poster session

Imagine that you are already at the conference. If you are just starting out on your poster-presenting career, it can be quite daunting. The answer is to be clear about how the session is likely to run and to be prepared for all eventualities.

Check where and when your poster will be displayed

You will have to arrive at the conference in time to hang your poster, or you must arrange for a colleague to do it for you.

Check your poster number

You will usually be told your poster number in advance so that you know where you should hang your poster. Remember to save this information – it is quite easy to find yourself at the poster session without your abstract book and no idea where to hang your poster.

Your number should usually be displayed on your poster

The poster number should be visible to delegates – those searching for a particular poster might be looking just for the number. Poster authors are often asked to either print the poster number on the poster or to leave a space for it to be stuck on. The guidelines for poster authors may tell you where your poster number should appear, but if not, the top left corner of your poster is a good spot.

Decide how you are going to attach your poster to the board

Organisers will often tell you how they would like you to do this. If you are not sure, make sure that you take pins, double-sided sticky tape or hook-and-loop tape with you. To avoid security problems, pack pins in your hold baggage if you are going on a flight. Sometimes there are emergency supplies of pins or sticky tape available to delegates who are struggling to attach their posters. This cannot be guaranteed, so it is your responsibility to be prepared.

Make sure your method of attachment is robust

Whichever method you use to hang your poster on the board, make sure that it is strong. Your poster may have an annoying tendency to roll up and spring away from the board after its long incarceration in a poster tube. Furthermore, people may brush against your poster, which could detach it from its fixings.

Check whether you need to be present in person at fixed times

Some conferences request that poster presenters are available next to their poster at particular times – often during breaks from the main conference sessions. This gives people a chance to ask you questions. It also gives you the opportunity to rendezvous with old friends and make new and potentially useful contacts.

Remember that you might have to give a mini-presentation of your poster . . .

Many large conferences now ask poster presenters to stand by their posters and give a mini-presentation, talking delegates through the data. If you have to do this, prepare notes and learn them before the conference starts.

. . . Or a mini-slideshow

Some conferences also allow a short PowerPoint presentation (three slides). If you are given the opportunity to do this, write the slides at the same time as you write the poster, and make sure that any changes you make to the poster are also made on the slides.

. . . Or to participate in a 'poster walk'

At some conferences, an expert in the field will walk around posters displayed in a given session and discuss them with interested conference participants. You should always make sure you are available for a poster walk that involves your poster so that you can add extra information (or defend it if necessary!).

Check whether there is a prize being given for the best poster

Why not go for the prize? It will look good on your curriculum vitae. Plan to attend the prize-giving ceremony anyway. It will give you an idea of the judges' criteria for a good poster. This will help you improve your poster writing and may help you to win the prize next year.

Ask for help from other people

You will be surprised how fast a conference creeps up on you when you are busy at work. There are several phases of poster development that involve other people. Find out who those people are and book their time so that your poster is produced well in advance of the conference. You do not want to be wondering where your poster is on the day that you travel to the meeting. You may need the services of the following people:

- *a scientific reviewer* to check the content; this will usually be one of your co-authors, PhD supervisor or boss
- *a translator* (if you are writing in your own language and translating into the language of the conference)
- *an 'editor'* – a colleague, friend or professional editor who can check your language and help you to proofread; this is not necessarily the same person as the scientific reviewer
- *a professional poster production company or graphic designer* (if you are not going to do the layout yourself)
- *a printer* – your institution's reprographics department or a commercial printer/copy shop
- *a courier* (if you are not carrying the poster to the conference yourself)
- *a travel agent* (if you need tickets booked; don't forget to book your travel, even if the conference is in your own country).

Develop a schedule

Get a calendar and work backwards from the date you leave for the conference. Give yourself plenty of time for each stage of the project. Make sure that you stick to the elements of the schedule that are in your control, even if others do not.

You may need several weeks to develop the perfect poster

Your schedule needs to allow time for:

- finalising data (pick a date and get all analyses finished by then)
- planning and devising illustrations (choose your design template, colours and illustrations and create high-quality photos)
- writing (if you are starting from nothing, a good guideline would be to give yourself 3 working days with no interruptions – you rarely get this sort of free time all at once, so plan a couple of weeks for writing)
- friendly review (get a friend to read it for sense and any major errors of science or language)
- academic review (get a supervisor or senior colleague to read it for scientific content and sense)
- revision and editing
- layout
- proofreading
- simultaneous friendly review and academic review of layout
- revision of layout
- final error-check of layout
- printing the poster to full size (this should only take a day, but it can sometimes prove tricky to print from PowerPoint, and highly coloured backgrounds may take quite a long time to dry after printing)
- checking the printed poster (allow time for reprinting if something is wrong on the first version)
- assembling materials for the conference (packaging the poster for transport, obtaining A3 handouts of the poster and packaging these for transport, packing pins/sticky tape/hook-and-loop tape).

Select your poster design software

Many scientific institutions routinely develop scientific posters in PowerPoint. Will you be doing the same? Do you know how? If not, get training as soon as possible. Alternative programs for developing posters are Illustrator, InDesign, LaTeX, PageMaker, Canvas and CorelDRAW. Any of these is suitable, but make sure you know how to use the program that you choose and that the people printing your poster can use the output from it.

If you are using PowerPoint, a pre-prepared template can save time and give a professional-looking result

There is no need to start from first principles – many pre-prepared PowerPoint poster templates are available, either from your institution or online. For more information on PowerPoint templates for scientific posters, *see* Chapter 8.

Decide which software you will use to draw graphs and other illustrations

Do you know how to use the software you have chosen? If not, get training as soon as possible. Simple bar charts and line graphs can be drawn in Excel or directly in PowerPoint. Many data-management systems (e.g. GraphPad Prism) allow you to draw more complex graphs. However, the output from some software packages may not be suitable for manipulation within PowerPoint, so give yourself time to redraw these graphs if necessary.

Find out whether your institution can print posters in-house or whether you will have to use an external printer

Some universities have reprographics departments that will print an A0 poster. Otherwise, you will have to have it printed externally. Most copy-shops have this facility, but it is wise to get recommendations from colleagues and to choose one that has experience in printing scientific posters.

Check who will pay for poster production

You must remember to check whether the cost of poster production is covered by your research grant or whether you have to pay for it yourself. If your institution does pay, check if it does so directly or whether you will you need to pay and claim it back.

Most posters are useful for the lifetime of the conference only

Normally, your poster ceases to be available to the scientific community after the meeting (and therefore cannot be cited as a reference). A few large conferences publish posters on a CD after the meeting or make electronic copies of posters available on the conference website.

A conference poster does not constitute 'prior publication' . . .

Just as for a conference abstract, presentation of data on a poster to people attending a conference does not adversely affect subsequent publication in a learned journal.

. . . But be careful of posters placed in the public domain

Occasionally, conference programme committees may ask permission to publish posters on a website, CD or even in a booklet to be made available after the meeting. This might be construed by a journal as 'prior publication'. If this happens, check with the journal in which you plan to publish your full paper. And if in doubt, say 'No'!

Decide on the objectives for your poster

Before you start writing and designing your poster, you should decide what you want to achieve at the conference. You might have more than one objective, for example to:

- publicise results
- generate discussion
- introduce your data to a new section of the scientific community
- encourage new investigators to join your project
- meet potential colleagues / collaborators
- promote your institution or project
- 'stake a claim' to an original research idea before competitors do so
- impress potential employers
- meet the requirement of your funding agency or other sponsors.

When you write and design your poster, keep your objectives in mind

For example, if your work is controversial and you want to stimulate debate, use headings that illustrate the controversy and make sure there is plenty of room for discussion. If you want to promote your institution, make sure that the logo features prominently in the top right corner of the poster, and devote a couple of lines of text to the excellent research being carried out within that institution.

Design your poster to attract and hold an audience

Some of the work in attracting an audience has already been done – let us assume you have an eye-catching and interesting abstract published in the abstract book, and you submitted your abstract with a good selection of key words. If the conference has an electronic conference programme planning service, these key words will bring your poster to the attention of delegates who are planning their poster viewing systematically using the abstract book. However, some people will simply wander around looking for interesting posters. A well-designed poster with an eye-catching title can help to attract an audience and hold their attention once they have arrived.

Write for the audience you want to reach

You cannot use the same scientific content and writing style for every audience. For example, your data may be relevant to both clinicians and pharmacokineticists, but these two groups will have very different interests. Before you begin to write, be sure that you understand the needs of the delegates at the conference that you are attending.

Decide on the 'take-home' messages you want to give your readers . . .

What level of scientific detail is appropriate? For example, are your illustrations too complex for this audience? Do you need additional discussion to make the relevance of your data clear?

. . . But make posters easy to read, regardless of the audience

You can use good poster design principles for any audience. It is courteous to everyone to make reading and assessing the poster as simple and pleasant as possible. No one, however motivated, wants to spend any more time trying to read and understand your poster than is strictly necessary.

7

Typography, headings and bullet points

You can enhance the attractiveness and readability of your poster with careful use of typography – the font you choose, the font size and additional features such as the use of bold or colour. Generally speaking, you get a better effect through being restrained and consistent in your choice of fonts and the additional effects that you employ. The headings you choose will help guide people through your poster and can provide a fast track to key data. Appendix 3 gives examples of styles for headings, text, and figure and table captions.

Choose simple fonts to enhance readability

Plain fonts are best, such as Arial, Helvetica, Times New Roman and Univers. Fonts have 'personalities', and some personalities may not create the right impression. For example, Comic Sans (the font that looks as if it was printed neatly by hand) is actually very readable but is perceived as informal – perhaps too informal for science.

Keep the body text simple and free of special effects

The body text should be the same size (at least 24 pt) and font style and use the same line spacing throughout. Limit the use of italics, bold and capitals to areas where they have scientific relevance, e.g. Latin names of organisms or abbreviations such as DNA.

Do not use more than two fonts in one poster

You can make a perfectly good poster with just one font, but if you do want more, two fonts are enough. Sometimes a sans-serif font such as Arial combines well with a serif font such as Times New Roman. You could use one for the body text and one for the headings. Don't forget that additional variety can be obtained through the size of the font and the use of bold, colour, or light-on-dark (i.e. 'reversed-out') text for headings.

Select font sizes carefully

Posters must be legible from a reading distance of 1–2 metres. If the font size is too small, people will have to get very close to the poster to read it, which will block the view of other delegates. If the font size is too large, people will have to stand a long way back, and there may not be room in the crowded poster hall. The minimum on-screen font sizes of the various parts of your poster are:

- title – 72 pt (96 pt is better)
- authors and affiliations – 56 pt
- section headings – 36 pt
- body text – 24 pt
- figure and table captions – 20 pt.

Do not go below 24 pt for body text

If you can't fit in all your text using 24 pt, resist the urge to reduce the point size. Cut the amount of text instead.

Make your main title easily visible from a distance

You can use font style, font size (72–96 pt), colour and space around the title to make it eye-catching. Black or dark blue lettering on a white background stands out well at a distance.

You may not need to make the title font bold if the font is already 'condensed'

If you are using a condensed font such as Arial Black in a title, do not add a further 'bold' command. This will squash all the letters together and make the text difficult to read.

You do not have to use title case in your title . . .

People often assume that the title of their poster has to be in title case, i.e. with all 'important' words capitalised, excluding 'small' words such as 'and' and 'in'. Although you can use title case in your main title if you really like the appearance of it, there can be problems. For example, the typographical conventions regarding which words should be capitalised in title case are somewhat obscure and may conflict with correct technical usage – for example, what would you do about the Latin name of an organism such as *Clostridium difficile*? Sentence case (only capitalising the first letter, proper nouns and anything else that should be capitalised for technical reasons) is easy and will not cause any problems.

. . . And you should avoid title case in headings or subheadings

Research suggests that headings and subheadings are easier to read if they are in sentence case rather than in title case. Furthermore, they often contain technical terms that may look odd with a capital letter.

Avoid using fully capitalised titles, headings and subheadings

CAPITALS ARE DIFFICULT TO READ IN LARGE QUANTITIES. They make it seem as though you are shouting, and it is very difficult to spot spelling errors. Furthermore, you cannot then use capitals correctly in Latin names of organisms, in acronyms or in other technical uses. Titles in all-capitals take up much more space and may cause your title or section heading to run on to more than two lines. You can make titles and section headings stand out very well without the excessive use of capitals.

Use capitals for abbreviations and acronyms

Abbreviations (e.g. DNA, MRI) and acronyms (names of clinical trials etc.) should be capitalised in titles, as elsewhere in your poster.

Avoid using *italics* for headings

Italics do not stand out particularly well in headings. It is simplest if they are restricted to use in scientific naming conventions (e.g. Latin names of organisms, genes and alleles).

Avoid WordArt and special text effects for titles and subheadings

WordArt does not usually enhance the appearance or readability of headings and may print differently from the way you expect. Other special text effects such as shadows may also print strangely and are seldom necessary. If you think you need a shadow behind your text, ask yourself why. Is it because the colour is too pale (in which case you could use a darker colour) or not bold enough (in which case you could use a larger point size)?

Use section headings to lead the reader through the poster

Headings are used to help readers move swiftly to their main areas of interest. In most scientific posters, the standard section headings are 'Objectives', 'Materials and methods', 'Results' and 'Conclusions'. However other sections, such as 'Introduction' or 'Background', 'Discussion' and 'Further information' may be appropriate.

Decide whether your title and section headings are to be centred or left-aligned

Titles and section headings can be centred or left-aligned. In the case of the section headings, it is important to be consistent – you can end up with some left-aligned within their columns and others centred, which will give your poster a messy appearance. In general, left-aligned section headings make it easier to ensure consistency and have a clean modern look. However, poster titles may be best centred if you also have to accommodate logos and a poster number in the banner section of your poster.

Keep section headings to one or two lines

Most section headings should be no more than one line long – you may need to edit out unnecessary words to achieve this. If absolutely necessary, a section heading may occupy two lines, as long as every heading is not like this. If a heading has just one or two words running on to a second line, look to see whether you can shorten it to one line by careful editing. Note that no full stops are needed at the end of headings.

Section headings should clearly separate areas of text

The headings of major sections, e.g. 'Results', should be large and bold (about 50% larger than the body text; a minimum of 36 pt versus 24 pt). To make section headings stand out even further, try:

- using white space above and below headings (not too much below or it will separate the heading from the body text)
- putting dark headings into pale-coloured bars (make sure these go all the way across the column even if not filled by text, otherwise you will create an inconsistent visual look)
- putting white or light headings into dark-coloured bars (these are known as reversed-out headings).

Consider the use of less formal section headings . . .

If it does not suit you, there is no need to use the standard 'Objectives', 'Methods', 'Results' and 'Conclusions' section headings you would use in a paper. You may choose to break your poster up into convenient sections that use more informative and informal headings, for example:

- instead of 'Objectives', you could have *'Does a high-protein diet increase exercise capacity in gerbils?'*
- instead of one big 'Methods' section, you could have *'Methods: selection of animals'*; *'Methods: diet'*; *'Methods: measurement of exercise capacity'*
- instead of one big 'Results' section, you could have: *'Results: body weight'*; *'Results: exercise capacity'*.

. . . And headings that state a result

If you have a clear-cut result, there is no reason why you should not state it in a heading and then explain the result in bullet points underneath. This type of heading is called a 'declarative' heading. An example would be *'Exercise capacity increased in males only'*.

Figure captions can state a result too

If you want to be a bit more positive about your results, you can also state a result in a figure caption. For example, your caption could say *'After 5 weeks, exercise capacity doubled in gerbils fed a high-protein diet'*, rather than *'Effect of diet on exercise capacity in gerbils'*.

Subheadings can help the flow within sections

Ideally, each section of your poster will have only minimal amounts of text, which would not require subheadings. However, if this is not possible, you might need subheadings to break up blocks of text and to aid understanding. Subheadings should be bold and in the same typeface as the body text of the poster. They can be the same size as the body text or slightly larger. As with the main headings, a little white space above and below subheadings can help them to stand out.

Put most of the body text in bullet points

Posters usually work better if you use bullet points rather than paragraphs for the body text. This isn't an absolute rule, however – if you have very small sections of text you may not need bullets.

Think twice if you have more than seven bullet points in a list

If you have a very long list of bullet points, it will be hard for people to follow the thread of your explanation – and it probably means that there is too much text in that section of your poster. To make life easier for your readers, you can consider:
- deleting some of the text altogether – do you really need it?
- subdividing the lists of bullets with section headings or subheadings.

Avoid sub-bullets unless absolutely necessary

Although programs such as PowerPoint make it easy to insert sub-bullets – and even sub-sub-bullets – these are seldom really needed. The extra indents waste space, make columns too long and create an ugly 'zig-zag' left-hand margin. If you find yourself with a bullet that has only one sub-bullet, the sub-bullet is almost certainly unnecessary.

Size bullets proportionally to the size of the text

Check to see how the bullets look in relation to the text size – normally the point size should be about the same.

Make sure that text associated with bullets is indented consistently

- It is usually better if the bullets themselves are flush left to the edge of the column, as in this example.
- There should be a consistent gap between each bullet and its associated text – if necessary, adjust this manually.
- If the text runs on to more than one line, make sure that all the text is indented – as in this bullet point.

Choose consistent symbols for bullets . . .

Do not suddenly switch from circles to squares – make the type and size of bullets consistent throughout the poster.

. . . And avoid 'novelty' bullets

While it may be very tempting to try to make your poster interesting with 'novelty' bullets, this can simply seem silly – assuming anyone notices them. Mouse- or heart-shaped bullets do not add to your scientific credibility.

8

Poster design and layout

Imagine yourself as a delegate at the conference. You have just an hour to look at all the posters in this poster session. What is going to make you stop and take the time to read *this* poster? Your reader needs to be able to get the most information from the poster in the shortest time, so a good design and layout are important for attracting and retaining attention of passing delegates.

You can use a PowerPoint poster template to save time and give professional results . . .

PowerPoint scientific poster templates are available, and these can be adapted to suit most needs. Unless you are particularly adept at graphic design, they will usually give a more professional result than trying to make all the decisions yourself about matters such as columns, fonts and colours. Note that by 'PowerPoint poster template' we mean a standardised layout designed specifically for making scientific posters, rather than the usual PowerPoint templates for making presentation slides.

. . . But it is fine to use any other design software

It is completely acceptable to design your own poster layout using any standard design software. However, you should still follow the principles laid out here for good poster design.

Check whether your institution already has a PowerPoint poster template with set colours and logos

You may be surprised to find that someone has already done a lot of the work for you and has designed an institutional template. It may even be compulsory to use such a template. If the template is compulsory, check to what extent it is permissible to change the layout and colours or move logos around.

If you have no institutional template, you can get a PowerPoint template from a colleague or from the Internet

Many websites provide PowerPoint poster templates. Some are better than others. Be sure that the PowerPoint template you choose follows the rules for good design – if not, adapt it so that it does. *See* Appendices 4 and 5 for examples of PowerPoint poster templates. Here are some websites that provide templates:

- www.radcliffe-oxford.com/biomedicine
- www.swarthmore.edu/NatSci/cpurrin1/postertemplate2.ppt#256,1,Slide 1
- www.posterpresentations.com/html/free_poster_templates.html
- http://teaching.ucdavis.edu/poster/template.htm
- http://miu.med.unsw.edu.au/downloads.htm#Scientific%20poster%20templates
- http://office.microsoft.com/en-us/templates/TC100214271033.aspx?pid=CT101439301033&WT.mc_id=42
- www.genigraphics.com/other/poster_templates.asp
- www.umiacs.umd.edu/~nedwards/documents/NCI_CPTI_2007_poster.ppt#256,1,Slide 1
- http://cf.ccmr.cornell.edu/templates/2003-Poster-Template.ppt#256,1,Slide 1
- www.studentposters.co.uk/templates.html

Read the instructions for use of each template

All templates differ slightly from one another. In particular, pay attention to any instructions for setting up page size and margins and how to insert illustrations.

If you are using PowerPoint, format your template for printing before you start

In PowerPoint you will really be making just one big slide. First format the slide so that it can be printed at A0 (the most common poster size and the maximum that PowerPoint can achieve). In PowerPoint 2007, choose 'Design' then 'Page Setup'.

Under 'Slides sized for:' choose 'Custom' and then set the page size to the same size that you want your poster to be (i.e. 84 cm wide × 119 cm high for A0 portrait and 84 cm high × 119 wide for A0 landscape). If the printed poster size needs to be bigger than A0, you will need to set the page size to half of the required final size and then enlarge it by 200% at the print stage. Beware: if you change the page size after finalising the layout, check the entire poster very carefully, as your layout may have changed.

Most layouts use columns . . .

Most templates are created using a layout with columns. In general, landscape posters work best with three or four columns and portrait posters suit two or three. Keep all columns the same width, as this helps readability. Variations in column width can make your poster look messy.

. . . But if you are experienced in graphic design, be creative

If you enjoy layout and design, you may choose to make your poster stand out from the crowd by creating a unique design, perhaps without columns. If you choose to do this, ensure that your information works effectively within the design and that you have not made the reader's task harder in your quest to be different. Good examples of creatively designed posters are shown in Appendices 6 and 7.

Aim for flow

Place the main elements on the page so that they are large enough to read easily and your eye flows from one to another. Readers usually expect to start somewhere near the top left of the poster and exit at the bottom right, though you can direct their eyes towards key areas with design devices such as colour and interesting graphics. Most people create flow by placing text, graphs and tables in a pleasing manner within a columnar format. Don't be tempted to put vertical dividing lines between columns; just leave this area as white space – it is easier to read, and vertical lines disrupt flow.

Give design emphasis to particularly important data

If you have one main scientific finding, put this in an obvious position. Visually, the top right of the poster is a 'hot spot' and the bottom left is a 'dead spot'. Consider how best you can emphasise the data. Can it be larger, more colourful, more unusual/special or darker than the rest of the poster? If you are using a template with columns, you can run particularly important graphs, photos or tables across two columns.

Place graphs, tables, photos and diagrams onto the page first

Put all graphs, tables, photos and diagrams onto the page in a logical manner and in a pleasing layout. Now look at the space that is left. Assess how much room there is for text and how much would look best as empty ('white') space. If you find this difficult to visualise on screen, try making a rough plan with pieces of paper laid out in a jigsaw on your desk.

Write your text to fill the areas not occupied by figures and tables

It is much easier to write to fill the available space than it is to carefully craft enough text to fill a whole poster and then to have to cut most of it out due to lack of space. To calculate the number of words that you need to write, simply put 'rubbish' text into text boxes above and below your figures and tables and count the number of words available to you. Many designers use 'Lorem Ipsum' dummy text to do this (there are Lorem Ipsum generators available on the Internet). Do not forget to replace the rubbish text with real text before you print your poster!

'White' or empty space is as important as the text

Add 'breathing space' around the text to avoid overcrowding and the possibility of one section accidentally merging with another. A good balance of elements for most posters is 30% text, 30% illustrations/graphs/tables/photos and 40% space. Sometimes 20% text, 30% pictures and 50% space is appropriate.

Fill the entire poster area evenly

Do not put all the information in the first couple of columns and have inches of white space at the end of the final column. An uneven design is less pleasing to read than a well-balanced one. Note that 'balanced' does not have to mean 'symmetrical' – asymmetrical designs can be very appealing. In general, people look to the right-hand side of the poster to find the conclusions. If you have not placed them there, make it very easy for the reader to spot them. Beware of large vertical posters . . . your conclusions section could end up at floor level!

Look out for 'widows and orphans' on your layout

A widow is a word or a few words that appear at the top of a column but belong with the paragraph at the bottom of the previous column. An orphan is the first line of a paragraph appearing at the bottom of a column with the rest of the paragraph continuing at the top of the next column. An orphan can also be a heading that appears at the bottom of a column without at least two or three lines of the following text. You can also get widows and orphans when a word or two from a block of text that flows around a figure or table become 'stranded' above or below the illustration. Widows and orphans look odd and reduce the readability of your text, so edit your layout to avoid these.

Use your design software tools to help with onscreen formatting

The tips given here assume that you will be working in PowerPoint 2007. However, other versions of PowerPoint and other design programs have similar functionality.

Set 2 cm margins at the edges of your poster

Do not allow text or pictures to hang over the edge of the on-screen slide or they will be lost in the final poster. Use the guide rulers within PowerPoint to set 2 cm margins around all sides of the poster, and keep all content within them. This will prevent data being lost if the poster is cropped to size at the printer.

Use gridlines and rulers for accurate alignment

In most PowerPoint poster templates, columns are set up using drawing guides, and then text boxes are placed within the guidelines. Make sure that you display the on-screen drawing guides (in PowerPoint 2007, on the 'Home' tab, in the 'Drawing' group, click 'Arrange', 'Align', and then tick 'Grid Settings', 'Display grid on screen' and 'Display drawing guides on screen'). For rulers, go to the 'View' tab, then 'Ruler' to help you with layout and alignment.

Turn on the spelling and grammar checker

PowerPoint has its own spelling checker (in PowerPoint 2007, go to 'Review', then 'Spelling'). This provides a useful first indication that your text is correct. Do not rely on the software totally, however; it is not a replacement for careful proofreading and editing.

For unjustified text, set text formatting to 'left-aligned'

To align your text at the left only, set the text formatting within PowerPoint to 'left-aligned' (in PowerPoint 2007, go to the 'Home' tab, 'Paragraph' and then 'Align left').

Check that the line spacing is consistent from one text box to another

Single-line spacing is usually enough, with double-line spacing between blocks of text (to set line spacing in PowerPoint 2007, go to 'Home', 'Paragraph', then 'Line spacing').

Create indented text manually

PowerPoint is not good at making consistent indents (tabs) – you may need to set the indents manually using the ruler (in PowerPoint 2007, go to 'View', then 'Ruler').

Take care with special symbols

Special symbols (for example, $\geq$, $\leq$, $\pm$, ®) that you added to your text in your word processing package may be lost in the transfer into PowerPoint or any other design package. Sometimes a useful little square appears to show you that something is missing – but not always! Check that all your special symbols are present. If you find an extra space in a sentence, ask yourself if a symbol has gone missing before you delete the space. You can insert special symbols within PowerPoint (in PowerPoint 2007, go to 'Insert' tab, then 'Symbol').

Turn off automatic hyphenation

Many software packages automatically hyphenate long words to make them fit neatly onto lines. However, allowing a computer to hyphenate scientific terminology can result in awkward and sometimes incorrect word breaks that reduce readability.

9

Colour and backgrounds for your poster

One of the good things about a poster is that it allows you to use colour to show your data to best advantage. Colour can also be used to make your poster more attention-grabbing. Unfortunately, inappropriate use of colour and background effects can also detract from the readability of your poster. So here are a few tips to help you use them appropriately.

Use a simple but attractive overall poster style

A well-designed poster has a uniform style of graphics, typeface and visually appealing colours. Avoid WordArt, semitransparent fills or textured backgrounds; although these may look fine on your computer, they detract from your data and may not print as expected. Clip art has no place on a serious scientific poster.

Make the background clean and subtle

Avoid busy, distracting backgrounds that can make the text more difficult to read. Usually, you should resist the temptation to make your poster pretty with a faded photo or picture in the background. This often seems like a good idea at the time, but proves difficult to put into practice if it clashes with numerous areas of text and illustrations.

Light-coloured backgrounds are best – and there is nothing wrong with white

Light-coloured backgrounds are least likely to lead to clashes with the text and illustrations, and they can add visual appeal. There is nothing wrong with a white background, especially if you have many other colourful items on your poster.

Avoid very dark or brightly coloured backgrounds

Very dark backgrounds can provide too much contrast with light text boxes, which will detract from readability. Very dark backgrounds can also prove difficult to print evenly. Very bright backgrounds, e.g. bright red or yellow, should also be avoided – they may attract attention but are stressful for readers to look at. Dark backgrounds also use a lot of ink, which can make your poster expensive to print.

Think carefully about your use of colour

PowerPoint and other electronic design packages give you the freedom to have unlimited colour on your poster. However, before you create a rainbow-coloured poster, it is worth thinking of the effects of colour on the reader. Too much colour can be just as confusing as too much text.

Check whether your institution or company requires you to use specific colours

Some institutions and companies require you to use specific background and accent colours to 'brand' the poster. Check whether this is the case for your poster, and if so, find out exactly which colours are specified.

You cannot expect everyone to like your choice of colours, but consider others' opinions

Colour preference is a very individual thing, and there are also strong cultural influences on how we react to colour. You cannot expect everyone to like your choice of colours, but if all your colleagues react strongly against your colours when you show them your draft poster, you may have made the wrong choices and need to think again.

Use colours that make the poster visually appealing

Stick to clear, bright colours on your poster. Browns, maroons, muted greens and brownish yellows can be depressing and will make the poster less attractive to the reader. The only exceptions might be if the colour is very appropriate to your subject (perhaps brown for the ecology of a mudflat) or is a standard colour required by your company or university.

One theme colour plus an accent colour is usually enough

Choosing one theme colour for items such as the background and headings can give a unified professional look to your poster. You can then vary the theme colour by using it at different percentages or adding a percentage of black for a darker effect. You might want to use a second colour for accenting key items – headings or bullets, for example. Restrained use of colour for backgrounds and headings is especially important if your poster already has many brightly coloured illustrations.

Enhance the flow of your poster with colour

A graduated background colour from left to right on a landscape poster or top to bottom on a portrait poster will help to lead the reader's eye. But keep it subtle – this should be a subliminal effect. You could also use coloured arrows to lead the reader from one area of the poster to the next. Another way to lead the reader's eye is to have similarly coloured text boxes behind the objectives and conclusions sections.

Consider using background colour to attract attention to key sections

Readers' eyes tend to be drawn towards coloured areas, so if one part of your poster (e.g. the main results) is particularly important, you could subdivide the poster vertically or horizontally with two different backgrounds (e.g. white and a pastel tint). Check that the visual effect is pleasing and not confusing.

Use colour to help with readability

Black or dark text on a white or light-coloured background is easiest to read. To make section headings stand out, consider white text on a dark background. It may be helpful for the overall design to put coloured boxes behind areas of text. If you do this, keep the colours pale behind the text or you will compromise readability.

Be consistent with colour on graphs . . .

Pick one colour for your experimental agent and another for your control. Use these consistently in every line graph, bar chart or pie chart. This makes the differences between experimental and control groups stand out clearly on the poster. The experimental group should be the strongest colour on the poster.

. . . And use blocks of colour, not patterns and textures

Colour provides the visual distinction between the experimental and control groups. It is not necessary to use patterning (e.g. cross-hatching) on bar charts or to have different types of line (e.g. dotted, dashed) on line graphs. Using colours and patterns together will lessen the impact for the reader.

Do not use red and green as your main comparison colours

Some delegates will be red/green colour blind and will not be able to tell the difference between your experimental and control groups.

Do not use yellow on a white background

Yellow does not show up well against a white background, and it is often a difficult colour to print correctly. In general, avoid yellow for headings, captions and lines or bars on graphs.

10

Writing your poster: general guidelines

When you look at posters being presented at a scientific conference, you will see that there are as many approaches to writing a poster as there are scientists! However, it is also apparent that some posters are much easier to read and understand than others.

Remember that you are writing a poster, not a paper

Many scientists treat writing a poster in the same way as writing a paper for a journal – and include almost as much information. But this is a bad idea. Journal articles and posters have different dynamics and content. Abstracts, complex tables, statistical intricacies and extensive lists of references belong in a paper, not on your poster.

Think of your poster as a 'stretched abstract'

Don't hide your data behind reams of text. Think of your poster as a 'stretched abstract' rather than a 'mini-paper'. On the other hand, make sure you add some value to the poster in the form of graphs, pictures and tables. We have seen one or two posters at congresses where, for unknown reasons, the presenters have just stuck a giant enlargement of their abstract up on the wall. That is guaranteed to be disappointing to potential readers. Even if you have not got as much data as you expected, there is always something you can add to the abstract.

Do a first draft using a word processing package

It is very tempting, particularly if you are short of time, to try to write your poster directly onto a PowerPoint slide or other publishing software. This is quite difficult to do, as you cannot read the entire poster onscreen and you have to work at high magnification. It is much better to write using a word processing package. Only import your document into PowerPoint once the various elements are finalised.

Write for the reader

Many delegates at an international conference will not have English as their first language. It is courteous to these readers to ensure that the writing style is easy to understand, even if the science is complex.

Meet the needs of 'skimmers'

Many delegates will 'skim read' a poster before deciding to invest time and effort in reading it fully. They will look at the beginning and end of the key sections for information of interest. Write your poster to meet the needs of these 'skimmers'.

- Clearly state your objectives.
- Make it obvious that the experimental design is innovative (if it is!) and that it will lead to data that will meet the objectives.
- Make it clear which are the important elements of the results.
- Link your conclusions with your objectives to demonstrate how well you have thought through your experimental design.

Apply the '30-second rule'

Skimmers generally spend 30 seconds or less deciding whether to read the full poster. It is your job to write and design the poster to meet the needs of skimmers so that they are convinced to read your poster in more detail – or, just as usefully, to get the 'bottom line' and move on. Once you have created your first draft poster, do the skimming test.

- What stands out in 30 seconds in your document?
- Have you added interesting information to that given in the published abstract?
- Does the information that you have obtained from the 30-second test match your objectives for your poster?
- Have you created a poster that gives delegates the message that you want them to have about your research?

Take care over spelling and grammar

There is a temptation to think that, provided the science is correct and can be understood, the language and spelling are irrelevant. *This is not true.* When delegates read a poorly written poster, they subconsciously receive the message that the author is sloppy, unwilling to put in additional effort to achieve excellence and does not take care of small details. None of these is a good characteristic for a career scientist. Do not forget that potential employers will be reading your poster – try to impress on all levels.

Keep the poster short and simple . . .

Keep the content concise and avoid overloading the reader with information not directly relevant to your data. The poster is probably the only piece of scientific writing where bullet points are the best way to write text. If you are drafting your poster in a word processing package, write all of your text in a 12 pt font and use 1.5 line spacing. Add all your figures, tables and photos into the file, with a page for each. If the file length exceeds seven A4 printed pages, you probably have too much material.

. . . Though not everything should be short!

Think about your use of abbreviations. It is tempting to use as many abbreviations as possible to cram additional information onto your poster. Avoid using too many non-standard abbreviations, however, as this reduces readability.

Define your abbreviations

Define non-standard abbreviations the first time that they are used. You do not need to define common or SI abbreviations, such as DNA, RNA, MRI, kg, mL or L.

Include all the key elements of a poster . . .

Although most posters follow a traditional series of headings, remember that you don't have to stick to these – variations are possible, as explained in Chapter 7. The standard elements are:
- poster number
- title
- authors and affiliations
- objectives
- materials and methods (or participants and methods for studies on people)

- results (unless the poster is mainly about the setting up of a study)
- conclusions
- a footnote giving the name of the conference, the venue and the year.

... Plus any formal or institutional requirements

You may also need to include:

- a logo (of your university, company, research institute, hospital, sponsor or grant-awarding body, for example)
- acknowledgements
- a conflict of interest statement or statement on the role of the funding source (especially in industry-sponsored posters)
- an abstract (never put an abstract on a poster unless the guidelines require it, as it wastes valuable space and duplicates the content of the poster).

... Plus any optional elements you consider necessary

The following sections may be necessary on some (but not all) posters. If in doubt, do not include them.

- Introduction/background (keep it brief unless the poster is mainly about the rationale for a study).
- Discussion (this is seldom necessary).
- References or further reading.
- Further information.

11

Writing your poster: banner components

The 'banner' is the bit across the top of the poster where you put the title, authors and affiliations, poster number and often any logos you are required to use. This area is usually where readers look first, so it is worth giving it close attention.

Have an eye-catching banner design

Some conference delegates read the abstract book and select the posters that they will look at and only visit those. Others simply wander around the poster session, browsing for information. For both types of delegate, an eye-catching title and its associated graphics or logos on your well-designed poster are likely to attract attention.

Check whether you have to use an institutional template

Some institutions and companies have designed a standard banner for all their posters, complete with graphics, logos and specified fonts. You may be required to use a standard banner to make the poster easily recognisable as coming from your institution.

Make sure you include all relevant logos

If your institution or sponsor requires a logo on your poster, do not forget to add it. If you are working in a multi-institution collaboration or have more than one sponsor of a study, make sure you include all the relevant logos, or someone is bound to be offended!

Put the logo at the top of the poster (unless you put it at the bottom!)

Your institution or sponsor may have guidelines for the placement of the logo on the page; if so, follow them closely. Many suggest the top right-hand corner of the poster. If you place it there, make sure that the logo does not interfere with or overlap the title on your poster layout. If there are no rules, there is no barrier to placing the logo in any convenient spot (including the bottom of the poster).

Do not use low-resolution logos taken from web pages

Make sure that you have the latest version of the logo in a suitable format for use in PowerPoint and at a resolution suitable for printing and enlargement (over 300 dpi). All too often, authors 'cut and paste' low-resolution logos from their university's web pages, resulting in a fuzzy logo on the printed poster. Contact your university reprographics unit or your company's PR department for a high-resolution logo.

Remember that your poster title should be the same as that of your abstract

It is confusing for readers to see a poster with a title that is different from the one printed in the abstract book. So, when you submit the abstract, you need to be thoughtful about how the title would appear on a poster. For more information on how to write the title for your abstract so that it will work well on your poster, check the tips in Chapter 3.

Keep the title as short as possible

The title will be in a large bold font at the top of your poster. Too many words will result in a huge block of text, which will be difficult to read and will look overpowering on the design. It is important to include all the key elements in your title (*see* Chapter 3), but edit out all wasted words so that the title does not take up excessive space.

Try to keep the number of lines in your title to the minimum

Titles should be a maximum of two lines long. If you run over onto a third line by just a word or two, you can reduce the font size by a fraction of a point or stretch the placeholder containing the title just a little, and it will often fit.

You can save space by using well-known abbreviations in the title . . .

As mentioned in Chapter 3, using a well-known abbreviation such as DNA, PCR or HIV in the title can help to save space, if you are sure that all your readers will understand it. However, avoid using uncommon or invented abbreviations just to make the title fit.

. . . But spell out unfamiliar terms in full

In scientific writing, it is conventional to spell out an unfamiliar term in full the first time it is used and then put the abbreviation in brackets immediately afterwards. However, if you plan to spell out a long term in the title of a poster (because it is unfamiliar to your readers), use your common sense about whether you really need to also give the abbreviation in the title. If the extra characters needed for the abbreviation take up too much space, you could wait until the first time you mention the term in the text to give the abbreviated version in brackets.

Avoid subtitles to the main title if possible

A subtitle is simply a way of packing more information into the title. Ideally, you should be able to say everything you need in the main title. Occasionally subtitles are unavoidable, but if you include one it should be in smaller text underneath the main title.

Student posters may be an exception to the 'no humour' rule

In Chapter 3, we explained why the temptation to use a funny title should usually be resisted. However, funny titles for posters may be acceptable for student posters produced for internal workshops or as a training exercise. A couple of effective examples we have seen on student posters are *'Snap, crackle and pop: when arm wrestling goes wrong'* and *'Pain relief during labour – does hypnosis deliver?'*.

Take care over authors' names

Check the correct spelling of the names of all your co-authors. Misspelled names are discourteous to your colleagues. Moreover, it is possible that a delegate will do an internet search using your names – misspelled names may make this harder and the delegate is likely to lose interest.

Use the authors' full names whenever you can . . .

Use the full first name and surname of each author if possible. Try to avoid having the surname plus initials. There are instances where people publishing in the same field have the same surname and initial letter, even though they have different first names. Using the name in full makes it clear who did the work.

. . . But if you have to use authors' initials, be consistent

Decide whether you will include all initials or just the first initial for each author. Having all initials is preferable, because you make it as clear as possible which person you are referring to. Do not put full points after initials. This avoids technical editorial issues, such as whether or not to put full stops after the first initial for a hyphenated name. It also makes the names easier to type!

Put authors' names and contact details prominently under the title

Delegates at conferences are often as interested in which people and institutions are publishing as they are in the actual data. Make sure the names and abbreviated addresses of all authors are clear and correct.

Highlight the presenting author

Some conferences ask you to highlight the presenting author. You can do this by underlining the presenting author's name, making it bold, or putting an asterisk after it. If you use an asterisk, make sure that it is clear on the poster what the asterisk means.

Do not put scientific or clinical qualifications in the author list

It is not usually necessary to put 'Dr' or 'Professor' or 'MD' or 'PhD' in the author list. These simply take up space, make the author list hard to read and add little useful information. You may want to add qualifications if you are providing full contact details for the presenting author.

Put the author affiliations below the author names

One or more lines may be needed to give the author affiliations, which should be in smaller type than the author names. Footnote indicators can be used to show which authors come from which institutions.

Add detailed contact information for the presenting author

As the presenting author, you should give delegates every opportunity to contact you after the meeting. Add your full postal address, telephone number (including country code) and email address in a further information section or as a footnote. Do not make the text too small, as you want it to be legible on your A3 poster handouts.

Make sure your address and contact details are correct

Address details are common sources of errors, and sometimes these are omitted altogether. If there is no contact information or if there is incorrect information, how will interested scientists contact you? Read and proofread the contact details for the presenting author (you!) with as much care as the rest of the text. Misspellings could result in letters or emails being delayed or going astray altogether.

Keep the contact details for other authors brief

You do not need full postal addresses for each author; just name of institution, department, city and country is usually sufficient. If the name of the city or country is in the name of the institution, there is no need to repeat it.

Put the poster number in a prominent position . . .

Some conference guidelines tell you to add the poster number to your poster and others do not. However, it is a good idea to get into the habit of adding it because you have a permanent reminder of where to hang your poster when you get to the conference. The poster number should also be included when you cite your poster on your curriculum vitae.

. . . Such as the top left-hand corner of your poster

The poster number is useful but not critical information, so do not put it in a visual 'hot spot' (such as the top right-hand corner); reserve hot spots for data. The top left-hand corner is a good position for the poster number. Leave some space between the poster number and the title – you do not want to reduce the impact of the title.

12

Writing your poster: the main text

Although most posters should be dominated by visual material, some text is necessary. You will probably need to explain your objectives, methods and conclusions and guide people around the results shown in graphs, tables and photos. Appendix 3 gives examples of styles for poster headings, main text, and figure and table captions.

Only include the poster abstract if instructed to by the conference guidelines

The abstract that you submitted to the conference is already printed in the abstract book or on the conference CD. Do not repeat the abstract on your poster unless the conference guidelines ask you to. If you are asked to include an abstract, it should be identical to the one in the abstract book. If you make any changes to it at all, change the title to 'Revised abstract'. If you really want to add your abstract to a printed handout of your poster, you can always print it on the reverse side.

Consider whether you really need an introduction section . . .

It is not compulsory to have an introduction section on a poster. This section could also be called 'Background' or even something more informal such as 'The problem' or 'Why such-and-such is needed'. In general, if you are short of space, you can leave out the context-setting that you would include in a paper. Delegates coming to read your poster are most interested in your new findings – they probably already know the wider context, and many of them will be experts in the field. However, if your research area is new, your approach is innovative or your study is yet to start, then some description of the problem and the rationale for your proposed solution may be appropriate. Furthermore, if you have little data and need to fill space on your poster, a background section can help.

. . . And if you have one, keep it brief and focused

You only need two or three sentences (30–50 words) to provide the rationale for a study. Anything more than that and you are probably trying to put a very wide perspective into a very small poster.

If you have an introduction, use only essential references

Do not use the introduction section to demonstrate that you know the entire literature. Only add references that are directly relevant to the points that you are making. Use superscript numerals for references to save space.

Make your objectives clear

A section called something like 'Objectives', 'Aims' or 'Hypotheses' is essential. You need to tell your audience what you were trying to achieve. Try to keep the objectives specific, for example: *To identify the mechanism of gene X expression and its role in breast cancer* or *To validate method Y for the identification of bacteraemic pathogens*. Avoid very global statements, such as *To cure cancer*.

Keep the objectives section short

The objectives section should only contain one or two bullet points (the absolute maximum is three – remember that you have to report on each objective in the conclusions section). Do not use long sentences, as this will lessen their impact. Try to keep the objectives section to 75–100 words.

Highlight the objectives section

As the objective is a very important element of your poster, consider using large, bold type or putting the text into a coloured box.

Restrict the materials and methods section to essential details only

It is not possible fully to describe a scientific method in under 200 words, so you need to select only the information essential for understanding your results. No one is going to try to repeat the study based on the methods in a poster, and you will be at the meeting to discuss the methods further. Long lists of inclusion and exclusion criteria for a clinical trial or details of incubation procedures etc. are not relevant.

If possible, keep materials and methods to five or six bullet points

The materials and methods section should be short, unless, of course, the poster is primarily about the development of a method. If you are following an already published method, you can simply cite the original reference. Remember to take a photocopy of that reference to the conference so that you can refer to it.

Use subheadings to highlight different methods

If your poster describes the use of several experimental methods to address the same objective, make it clear which method is which. Divide the text using subheadings. If you do this, make sure that you use similar subheadings to divide the results section. That way delegates can quickly link a given method to its result.

A picture speaks a thousand words

It can be easiest to describe a technique or a protocol using flow charts, diagrams or photos. If you can provide an illustration to describe your methods, it is far preferable to writing detailed text.

The results section is the main part of your poster

Aim to provide a complete picture of your experimental results. Try to make this interesting by using a mix of text, graphs, tables and photos or other illustrations. Keep the text to the minimum needed to tell the story (200–300 words), either as sentences or bullet points.

Do not hide data in the text

All your data should be in the form of clear graphs, photos, tables, flow charts or diagrams. Your text should make a simple statement of the finding, with the actual data being presented visually.

A picture still speaks a thousand words in the results section

Unlike in scientific papers, there is no limit on visual material in a poster; you can have as many graphs, tables and photos as you need. However, do not overdo it. Try to ensure that there is a clear reason for the use of each visual item. Too many graphs can be as confusing as too much text.

Think about the best way to present your data . . .

In some cases there will be only one format for representation of data, e.g. survival curves. However, often you have several potential options. Think clearly about which option is best for your data.

. . . Such as frequency data

Consider a pie chart rather than a table. However, if you have to compare several sets of frequency data, it may in fact be better to use a table – it is difficult to compare one pie chart with another.

. . . Or discrete data points

Bar charts are ideal for this type of information. Think about whether the bars should be vertical or horizontal. Which would fit better onto the page?

. . . Or continuous data

For continuous data (relating to outcomes over time or over a dose range), line graphs are best. Try not to have more than four or five lines on a line graph if you want the reader to make comparisons. More than five lines are fine if you are simply trying to demonstrate that all the data are similar.

. . . Or audiovisual data

If your poster is all about the song of cicadas or communication between whales, consider letting the delegates hear your auditory data. If your poster is about real-time changes in cellular morphology, it would be nice to see a video of the cells changing shape. With the advent of tiny and relatively cheap MP3 players and similar devices, it is now simple to carry samples of your data with you to conferences. Some devices are small and cheap enough to attach to the poster board; delegates can press a button to hear or see your clip. Alternatively, you might want to take a laptop into the poster hall or even have relevant files on your mobile phone.

Graphs and photos have more impact than tables

Try to present your most important data as graphs – it is much easier to read and understand these from a distance. If you have to use a table, make sure that you highlight the areas of interest to make it easy for the reader.

Link your graphs, photos and tables to the text

To help your reader to follow the flow of your results, all graphs and tables should be cited and numbered in the text, e.g. Figure 1, Table 1. Where possible, the illustration should appear adjacent to where it is mentioned in the text. If readers have to search for the relevant information, they may get bored and move on to another poster.

Add a short explanatory caption to each figure or table

Each graph, table, photo or diagram should have an explanatory caption. Try for one or two lines of caption, with three as an absolute maximum. Choose a different size or style of font, or put captions within a box or reverse them out of a colour, so that figure or table captions cannot be confused with body text.

Keep figure and table captions consistent

Stick to one style of caption for figures and tables, and be consistent about where you place them. This will enable readers to move quickly and simply from one major result to another. If a figure or table occupies the whole width of a column, the captions should go consistently either above or below the figure or table. If a figure or table occupies only half the column width, the caption can usefully be placed to one side. Simply by reading the captions and looking at the figures and tables, a reader should be able to understand the main messages of your poster.

Do not be afraid to state a result in a figure or table caption

If it makes it easier for the reader, and you have a clear result, don't be afraid to state '*X reduced Y in Z*' in the figure or table caption, rather than just '*Effect of X on Y in Z*' (*see* Chapter 7).

Consider how graphs and tables will look at full poster size

Graphs and tables that look good on an A4 piece of paper may not look as impressive when they are enlarged to A0. All the data points will move away from each other on enlargement, and any white space will seem a lot more extensive. Think about how the data are represented – is it clear which value relates to the experimental agent and which to the comparator? Are significance values close to the data points or will they ultimately be floating around alone in a sea of white space?

Use headings to guide the reader through your results

If you are reporting the results from several different methods, use simple, short subheadings to make it clear which results are from which method. You can have subheadings that are statements of results. For example, *'For the primary endpoint, drug A is superior to drug B'* or *'MRI scanning clearly demonstrates the lesion'*. If your materials and methods section is divided by subheadings, mirror these in your results section.

Emphasise subheadings in your poster design

Make sure that there is a clear break between the end of one paragraph and the following subheading. Make use of bold fonts and white space above and below the heading. If the subheading is important, consider putting it in a coloured box.

The conclusions section is the most important part of your poster

Many delegates will look first at your conclusions to determine whether they will bother to read the rest of the poster. Only draw conclusions based on the data in your poster. You do not usually need to discuss the wider scientific context relating to your conclusions (if you really need to, you could do this in a brief discussion section). However, you may wish to mention any important implications or applications of your findings, or future work.

Check that your conclusions relate to your objectives

You should relate your conclusions to the study objectives and demonstrate how your research has met them (or not!). Each of your objectives should be addressed by the conclusions. If your data do not allow you to conclude anything relating to one of your objectives, consider removing that objective from the poster, or state why it could not be met.

Three or four bullet points in the conclusions section is optimal

You should highlight your key findings only – try to keep your conclusions to three or four main points. Some research suggests that, in English, readers find three points a satisfying and memorable way to summarise a story or answer a question. The final bullet point should be the major implication of the study, if there is one. Try to limit this section to about 150–200 words.

Highlight the conclusions section

As the conclusions section should relate directly to the objectives section, consider using the same large, bold type or coloured box that you used for the objectives. This will provide a visual link on the layout.

A discussion section is optional

In general, discussion is best reserved for full papers, as it is not possible to discuss an area fully in just a few words. For most posters, therefore, it is not necessary to include a discussion section, but if you feel that your data need explanation or to be set into a wider context, you might choose to include one. If you do include a discussion section, keep it short – about 100–150 words. To save space, use superscript numerals for references.

You can have a 'Future work' or 'Questions to be answered' section

Although mention of future work can often go in the conclusions section, sometimes it is helpful to put it in a separate section. This approach can be especially useful if you are part of the way through a long project and want to interest people in what you are planning to do next. But as in the abstract (*see* Chapter 4), resist the temptation to make vague statements like '*More studies are needed . . .*'.

13

Writing your poster: bits and pieces

In addition to the title, authors and main content with its figures and tables, you may want to include certain additional elements, such as references, acknowledgements and conflict of interest statements. These things may be necessary, but they are not very interesting to most readers (except those who are being acknowledged or referenced!). This chapter is about how to put these 'bits and pieces' into your poster without distracting your readers or wasting precious space.

Isolate uninteresting elements from the rest of your poster

One problem with putting the uninteresting but necessary information as the final item in your final column is that, if it comprises a lot of text, you can end up with a large box of boring information in the bottom right-hand corner, which is where most people will look for your conclusions. One way round this problem is to find some way of separating the boring information graphically from the rest of your poster. For example, you could draw a line right across the bottom and put all the boring information below this line in small type.

Keep references to a minimum . . .

You should only add references if you need to support statements in an introduction section or if you need to reference a specific method or support a conclusion. In most posters, introductory sections are unnecessary, so you may not need references at all.

However, all scientists are trained to reference documents, so the temptation is to sneak in a few references or add a further reading list. Avoid the temptation; abstracts and posters are exceptions to the referencing rule.

. . . And if you have to include references, limit them to four or five

You do not want to use up the valuable space on your poster by filling it up with references. Try to limit yourself to four or five. Think about where you will place the references on the final layout. You do not need to have the traditional references heading and section straight after the conclusions section. Consider running the references across the bottom of the poster.

Use a small font size . . .

Wherever you locate them, put the references in a small font size so that they do not take up too much space on the layout, but make sure that they will be legible on your A3 handouts.

. . . And keep citations short

Use superscript numerals to indicate references in the body of the text; this uses the minimum of space. In the references section, cite the references numerically in the order that they appear in the text. You do not need to type out the entire reference citation; including the title of the article can be a waste of space. Just give enough information so that someone else can find the reference – first author with initials, followed by *et al.*, the abbreviated journal title, year, volume number and page range.

Don't forget to cite yourself

If you do have a section that needs references, try to cite your own papers as well as those of others. This helps to establish your credentials in the field.

If you include references, ensure they are correct

It is really boring to type, edit and proofread references. However, your attention to detail might come into question if your references are full of typographical errors and different formats. Choose one reference style and stick to it. If you are unsure of the abbreviated journal name, check one of the online databases, such as PubMed, which uses the accepted abbreviations.

Think twice before adding a further reading list

You should only add a further reading list if you are doing such groundbreaking research that your readers are unlikely to know anything about your field. In general, further reading lists are redundant on posters.

Acknowledge practical and financial support

It is important to mention people and organisations that have supported you in the research reported in your poster. It is most likely that you will need to acknowledge the funding that you have received from the state, a charity or a commercial company. You may also want to acknowledge technical, statistical or editorial support from individuals not listed as authors on the poster. You do not necessarily need a formal acknowledgements section. You could put the acknowledgements under the references in a small font size across the bottom of the poster.

You may need a 'conflict of interest' statement

In some fields, especially drug trials, it is becoming customary to acknowledge any conflict of interest on posters, as would be done in published papers.

'Further information' is generally optional . . .

This section is usually optional, and should only be considered if you have plenty of room left on your poster layout once all the essential material has been added. You might decide to supply your full postal address and telephone number or your email address (if not included in the banner) or a website containing scientific information, such as extensive data tables or the statistical program that you used in the poster. You might also consider adding a link to an online .pdf version of your poster.

. . . But if it is essential, you can use a small font size

Sometimes it may be essential to include a further information section. If you are short of space, consider running the information across the bottom using a small font size.

Consider adding a footnote referencing the current conference

Somewhere on the poster, in small print, it is worth adding 'Presented at . . .' followed by the full name of the conference and the year. This may seem irrelevant on your first couple of posters, but when you have presented at many conferences, you will be glad of this reminder!

14

Tips for tables

Many posters will contain tables of data. These can be quite hard work to understand in a hurry, so here are a few tips to make them as simple as possible for your readers.

Make the table and its caption tell a self-contained story
Each table should deal with a specific aspect of the research question, representing just one key idea or message.

Keep tables simple and do not overwhelm readers with information
Most people (except your closest colleagues or competitors) will not have the time or patience to read very complex tables. Do not try to pack too much data into one table – you do not have to include every variable that you measured. Think about which data are really needed to make your point. Ideally, try to have no more than seven rows (including the header rows) and five columns in a table.

Use a figure in preference to a table
Readers of posters have little time to devote to reading your table, so it is usually better to use a figure if it would do the same job just as well. Research suggests that the average reader prefers information to be displayed graphically where possible.

Use a table where you need to show detailed numerical information . . .

There are times when readers need to see precise numbers or detailed statistical information, in which case a table allows you to compress a lot of information into a small space. However, you may also consider combining the best of both approaches by adding key values to line graphs and bar charts.

. . . Or to display discontinuous variables

Tables may be needed if you are comparing very different kinds of information between groups. For example, if you want to show baseline data, such as sex, age, weight, smoking history and concomitant diseases, for two groups of participants in a clinical trial, you will need a table.

Choose a consistent style for tables within the poster

In contrast to a scientific paper, where the journal dictates how to format tables, there is no standard format for tables in a poster. PowerPoint offers a wide variety of table styles that you can adapt to suit your needs. If you have several tables on the poster, they should have a similar appearance. Think about aspects such as the number, width and colour of lines; the width of columns and the depth of rows; whether you require vertical lines as well as horizontal lines; the fonts and type sizes used; and the colour and shading of the main row and column headings.

Do not import tables directly from word processing packages

Tables formatted beautifully in a word processing package often lose all their formatting and become difficult to manipulate when transferred directly into PowerPoint. It is usually best to create your table within PowerPoint if possible.

Do not 'cut and paste' tables from previous posters, PowerPoint slide sets or papers

Always create exactly the table that you need for this poster. Do not think 'Here's one I prepared earlier'. It is likely that the original will not be in the correct format for your poster, and is unlikely to contain exactly the data that you need to tell the story of the poster that you are writing today. Tables cut and pasted from .pdfs of papers are often blurred when imported into PowerPoint, so will affect the look of your poster.

Give each table an appropriate caption

Readers should be able to understand the table without looking at the main text of the poster. Often, the table caption will include important information such as independent and dependent variables and the material, species or patients studied. Thus a typical table caption might be '*Table 2. Effect of age, sex and nationality on poster design preferences of postgraduate students in a worldwide multicentre study*'.

Consider whether you can put some experimental methods into the table caption

Putting some of the experimental detail in the table caption rather than in the methods section may save space and make the table and its caption easier to understand as a self-contained unit. If you do this, make sure that your caption is no longer than three lines, or the reader may lose interest.

Keep the table layout clear and uncomplicated

Readers do not have much time to devote to each table on your poster, so it is important that they can find the main points as quickly as possible. Consider highlighting key points with colour or bold type.

Avoid too many gridlines

When you set up a table in PowerPoint, the default is to show all borders around individual cells. Too many lines distract the eye and make the table harder to read. Remove all but the most essential lines. In PowerPoint 2007, double-clicking on the table will bring up 'Table Tools'; you can then click on 'Design' and adjust the borders. The main horizontal lines should be at the top and bottom of the table and under the heading. It is often unnecessary to have vertical lines within the table (*see* Table 14.1, below), though you may decide to have lines at the extreme right and left of the table to make it into a box.

Distinguish row and column headings visually

There are many ways of making headings within a table stand out for ease of reading. For example, you could use bold type, a background colour, or light type on a dark background.

Keep column and row headings short

Think about the shortest form of words that you can use to prevent the table being unnecessarily wide. If needed, headings can occupy two lines.

Where applicable, column and row headings should include units of measure

Units of measure are usually given in brackets after the category, e.g. weight (kg). For SI units, there is no need to define abbreviations. However, any unusual abbreviations for units should be defined in a footnote underneath the table.

Align the column and row headings consistently

A common style is to align the row headings flush left and to centre the column headings. The contents of the columns are then aligned on the decimal point. However, it is also possible to left align both the column headings and the contents, especially if the contents are not numerical data, but words or symbols. Whichever system of alignment you choose, it is important to be consistent within and between tables. This makes the poster more visually pleasing and professional.

Numbers are normally aligned on the decimal point in a column

Thus, your table may look like this:

Table 14.1 Favourite hot drinks among postdoctoral researchers at three UK universities (data collected using the Beverage Research Questionnaire)

Favourite drink (% respondents)	Oxford	Cambridge	Manchester
Coffee	53.5	47.2	44.6
Tea	23.5	23.8	25.4
Chocolate*	15.1	29.0	26.0
Other[†]	7.9	0.0	4.0

*including cocoa;

[†]including milk (from any animal, or soy milk) and hot water

Did you notice something about this table, however? The data could just as easily have been displayed as 100% bars (*see* Chapter 16), which would be visually much more interesting.

Arrange tables so that important comparisons are made from left to right . . .

Most readers are accustomed to reading tables from left to right, not top to bottom. This makes the table easier to read and understand.

. . . And present experimental data followed by control data

If you are comparing an experimental dataset with controls, the convention is to put the experimental data first (in the left-hand columns) and the control second (right-hand columns). Make sure that you stick to this convention for all tables to help the reader quickly assess the information that you are presenting.

Give row headings and subheadings a logical order

Rather than just putting your row headings down in the order you first thought of them, think about what order will make the data easiest to interpret. If you have many row headings, grouping them will make the data easier to understand. For example:

Coffee
    Instant
    Filter
    Espresso
    Cappuccino
Tea
    Black
    Green
    Herbal

Indented subheadings can be difficult in PowerPoint

You cannot use tabs in PowerPoint to create standard indents. Avoid the temptation to use the space bar, as this can result in inconsistencies. Use the 'Ruler' function in PowerPoint to set a standard distance for each indent.

Use colour, shading or bold text to highlight key areas of the table

If the table is complex, consider emphasising the most important parts. For example, if your table has rows giving data for many outcomes or variables, you might want to highlight the most important by putting the numbers in bold or in a different colour or by applying a background tint to the whole row.

Choose units that take up as little space as possible

Think about which units of measure will make the most concise table. Choose units that eliminate unnecessary zeros – for example, 1.3 kg is better than 1300 g. Likewise, 13 mg is better than 0.013 g. However, it is also important for units to be consistent, so you may have to allow space to accommodate precise measurements that range from very large to very small. Consider rounding numbers up or down to make them simpler to understand.

Be consistent with decimal places . . .

Use the same number of decimal places in all values for one variable. Use the same number of decimal places in standard deviations, errors or confidence intervals as in the mean.

. . . And do not use excessive decimal places

Ask yourself how accurately you measured each variable, and do not give numbers down to several decimal places if it is not really relevant. For example, it is usually acceptable to give mean values rounded up or down to the same number of decimal places as the individual numbers used to calculate them.

Avoid irrelevant detail . . .

People will not have time to study all the data in your poster in detail, so consider simplifying the content to make it easier to understand. Not every variable you measured needs to be displayed.

. . . And information that does not aid understanding

For example, if you have demographic information, giving the percentage of male patients is sufficient. It can be assumed that the others were female!

Include standard deviations, confidence intervals and p values where appropriate

Include all the statistical information necessary to allow readers to draw appropriate conclusions about your data. You could give p values in a separate column or save space by using asterisks, which are then defined in footnotes. A standard series is $*p < 0.05$; $**p < 0.01$; $***p < 0.001$.

Make sure that columns of numbers add up correctly

Check that columns that are supposed to add up to 100% or the total sample size do so. If parts of the sample are missing for some reason, or if they appear in more than one place, explain this in a footnote.

Refer to your tables in the text

Even though your table and its caption form a self-contained self-explanatory unit, it is customary to refer to it in the text of the poster (e.g. Table 1). That way, if people are reading the text in detail, it will be easier for them to find the relevant table. Although tables should ideally be close to related text, layout considerations sometimes mean that they cannot be immediately adjacent.

Make sure all data given in tables coincide with values in the text

If any of the numbers in a table are mentioned in the text, they must match each other.

Think about whether you should give actual data as well as percentages . . .

Percentages help readers to make instant comparisons when the sample size varies between groups. However, many readers would like to know the actual numbers as well. If so, it is often best to give percentages with the actual numbers next to them in brackets in the same column, i.e. 50% (24/48).

. . . As percentages alone can be misleading

If you see a percentage value of 50%, you might have different views on the data if you discovered that this was 50% of a sample of two rather than 50% of a sample of 300.

Define any non-SI abbreviations or symbols used in footnotes

Readers do not want to search through your poster looking for the meaning of abbreviations, so it is usually best to define them in a footnote to the table. Footnotes can be in small type so that they do not spoil the overall look of the table or take up too much space.

Try to avoid leaving cells blank unless absolutely necessary

An empty cell in a table leaves the reader guessing; if the value is zero, put 0, or if you have no value for that cell, put a dash or an abbreviation (for example n.d. for not determined). Make sure that you define the abbreviation in a footnote.

Remember that wide tables can cross more than one column in your poster

If the table works best over one-and-a-bit columns, you could consider putting the legend beside it rather than above it.

15

Tips for graphs

Many posters will make use of graphs. The details of how these are constructed will depend on your data and the conventions of your own research discipline. However, here are some general principles for constructing effective graphs.

Remember that figures are often the first thing that readers look at

Many people are visual learners who will look first at your figures, hoping that they will tell them the most important results. So your graphs, charts and photos have to make a good first impression.

Select the simplest type of graph to represent your data

It is usually evident what type of graph you will need to display your data. However, you will often have the choice between simple and complex representations. For a poster, always choose the simplest graph that will do the job. Reserve complex diagrams for papers, where you have space to explain them fully.

If you use complex concepts, make sure that you understand them

If you are not an expert in data analysis and representation, you might like to ask a colleague who is expert in statistics about how best to represent complex data. Do not blindly accept their advice, however. Make sure that *you* understand what the resulting graph tells you – you do not want to be caught out struggling to explain your own data analysis to a conference delegate.

Use scatter plots for comparing two variables

A scatter plot compares two variables (e.g. weight and height). The individual data points are plotted and then a linear correlation coefficient is calculated or a regression line fitted. This gives a good visual picture of the relationship between the two variables.

Use line graphs for continuous data

Use line graphs where the independent variable (the X axis) is a measurement (i.e. is continuous). For example, you might be comparing the effects of two or more different treatments over time.

Create simple graphs in PowerPoint or Excel . . .

Simple line graphs and scatter plots can be generated within PowerPoint or Excel. Take care when you enter the data into the spreadsheets – a mistyped entry could alter your interpretation of the data.

. . . Or for more complex data, use a scientific graphics package

Some types of graph have specific structures (e.g. survival curves) that are difficult to reproduce in PowerPoint or Excel. For these you should use a graphics package with specific capability in the format that you require. When creating your poster, format the graph according to the style of your poster, then export the graphics file to an image file that you can import into PowerPoint. Check that all the data points and labels have survived the transition from graphics package to poster.

Choose scales so that your graph has pleasing proportions

The slope of the graph should not be excessively steep or shallow. Line graphs are comfortable to read if they are in 'landscape' format, i.e. if the length of the vertical (Y) axis is about two-thirds that of the horizontal (X) axis. For scatter plots, the axes should be the same length.

Plot the dependent variable on the Y axis and independent variable on the X axis

The usual convention is to put an independent continuous variable (e.g. time) on the X axis and a dependent continuous variable (e.g. a measure of treatment effect) on the Y axis.

Label each axis with what was measured . . .

It is surprising how often graphs, even in published papers, do not have the axes labelled clearly to indicate the variables that have been plotted. It is even more important on a poster to label the axes clearly, as there may be little supporting text to enable the reader to work it out (and they do not want to take the time to do so, anyway).

. . . And in the appropriate units

Choose units so that the graph will not distort the data. The scale points on each axis should usually have equal intervals (unless you are using a logarithmic scale). Use units that eliminate unnecessary zeros – in other words, 1.3 kg is usually better than 1300 g. If you use superscript numbers, check them very carefully, or 10^3 could mysteriously turn into 103.

Use units that everyone will understand

Some computer programs cannot handle superscripted numerals. Consequently, axis values on printouts may be non-standard. As the person handling the data, the output will be clear to you, but it may not be clear to a reader. If you mean 6×10^3 then change the axis labels to say that – do not be content with output such as 6E3 or 6\3.

Start the scale at zero – or if you do not, make this clear

You might be considered to be attempting to mislead readers if you exaggerate differences between groups by not starting your scale at zero. On the other hand, there may be good scientific reasons not to start at zero – for example, you are using logarithmic data or a clinical rating scale that does not have a zero category. If you break a scale or start beyond zero, make this clear with a cross-mark on the axis.

Use downward sloping lines on negative scales

If your data consist of negative values – for example, if you want to indicate a reduction in a particular variable – construct the graph with the X axis at the top instead of the bottom. Negative data will then be represented as downward sloping lines.

Be consistent with tick marks on your axes – they should be 'in' or 'out'

Tick marks (the little lines that indicate values on the X and Y axes) should all point in a consistent direction – either 'in' or 'out'.

Avoid excessive number labels on your axes

You do not have to have a number next to every tick mark, especially if that means that you would have to make the font size very small in order to fit all the numbers in. So do not forget that you can use unlabelled tick marks for subdivisions between labelled tick marks.

Make sure that tick marks line up with their number labels

Graphs created in PowerPoint and Excel sometimes appear with the numbers in between the tick marks on the axis, instead of aligned with the tick marks. This happens when the number is inadvertently treated by the program as a category, not a number. Check and change this if necessary.

Emphasise the data, not the axes

The graph lines are where you want the readers to look, so the thickness of these lines should be greater than that of the axes. Most scientific graphics programs will take care of this for you.

Do not extend axes too far beyond the data

The X and Y axes should extend only to the next tick mark on the axis after the maximum values for the data. Again, your graphics program will probably take care of this for you.

Do not try to fit too many lines on one graph

Think about how much information readers will be able to absorb. For example, line graphs with more than five lines may be too difficult to read, especially if the lines overlap. Of course, you should not omit scientifically relevant data simply because it looks ugly, but think about whether you are trying to show too many things on a single graph.

Colour helps your graph lines to stand out . . .

When devising graphs to be printed in black and white in papers, you may be used to using dashed or dotted patterns to distinguish between two or more lines. On posters, however, you can use colour, which usually makes life easier for your readers.

. . . But try to avoid using red and green lines together on the same line graph

Red-green colour blindness is quite common and might lead to confusion with some graphs. If this is a potential concern, you can use www.vischeck.com to check how your graphs would look to a colour-blind person.

. . . And do not use yellow for lines

Yellow does not show up clearly on a pale or white background, and it is a colour that is notoriously difficult for printers to get right.

Consider simply labelling lines rather than using keys

If colour keys are used, readers have to look in two different places to find out what is being compared on your line graph. If the graph is quite simple, why not label the lines themselves instead of using a key?

If you use a key, put it on the graph itself, not in the figure caption

Usually keys to symbols or lines should be generated as part of the graph rather than added later as part of the figure caption. This is for two reasons. Firstly, it is easier for readers to interpret keys if they are as close as possible to the data to which they refer. Secondly, if your graph was generated in one program and your caption in another, it may be hard to match the symbols and colours used on the graph with those in the caption.

Position the key to make the most of the space available

Although your graphics program may automatically place the key to one side of the graph, this may waste a lot of space. You can often make the 'working area' of the graph effectively larger if you put the key in any convenient empty area of the graph, rather than alongside it.

Add extra information to lines where necessary

You can help readers to understand your results by highlighting key points on your line graphs. For example, you can add p values at appropriate points to show differences between groups at specified time points. Or you might want to draw a horizontal line across the whole graph to indicate a normal or target value or a vertical line to indicate the time point at which two lines start to diverge.

Define any abbreviations used on the figure or in its caption

It is important to make graphs and their associated captions self-contained so that readers do not have to search the rest of the poster to discover what abbreviations mean. SI units and very common abbreviations need not be spelled out, but other abbreviations should be defined either in the key or figure captions. Be consistent from one graph to another in the abbreviations you use and where you define them.

Use consistent symbols from one graph to another . . .

Your graph may include data points marked with symbols, which should be consistent in colour and shape from one graph to the next. Using different symbols for the same group in two different graphs is potentially very confusing. Always define the meanings of symbols in the key.

. . . And use consistent colours

Make sure that data from your experimental group are represented in the same clear, bright colour on every graph. This will make your experimental data stand out on the poster. Do not use the same colour or colour tones for the control group, as it will be difficult for the reader to distinguish experimental and control at a glance.

p values are usually indicated with asterisks

It is standard practice to indicate statistically significant differences on graphs with one or more asterisks. The usual sequence is *$p<0.05$; **$p<0.01$; ***$p<0.001$. As with other symbols, define the meanings of asterisks on the graph or in the key.

Add error bars as appropriate

Error bars may be needed in some graphs. Make it clear in the key or figure caption what they represent (e.g. standard error, standard deviation or confidence intervals).

If you use someone else's published figure, always acknowledge the source . . .

Occasionally, it may be appropriate to include other people's data in your poster so that they can be compared with your own. If you reproduce a figure first given by another author in a paper, you must make this clear and include the reference. This is important as a courtesy to the original author – imagine how you would feel if someone included your figure in his or her poster and did not acknowledge it. An appropriate format might be 'Reproduced from . . .' or, if you changed it, 'Adapted from . . .'. If the data are taken from a published paper, there may be copyright issues (*see* below).

. . . But try to avoid just 'cutting and pasting' a graph from a .pdf

If you 'cut and paste' a graph from a .pdf of a paper, it will usually appear fuzzy when printed as part of your poster. It will also be in an inconsistent style and may only be in black and white when the rest of the poster is coloured. Ideally, you should redraw a figure from a published paper in the style of your poster and on the same scale as the rest of your graphs. This will allow direct comparison with your own data and will ensure that the graph prints clearly.

Be aware of copyright issues

Copyright laws vary from country to country, and we are not experts. Universities often have licence agreements covering the use of copyright materials for educational or research purposes, and you should check with your own institution. Generally speaking, it seems to be widely accepted that you can reproduce a figure from someone else's paper in a research poster *provided that you acknowledge the source*. The copyright situation is much more complicated regarding more permanent uses, e.g.

if your poster is placed on an institutional or commercial website or used for any commercial purpose. If in any doubt, check the regulations in your own country and write to the copyright holder (the journal and/or author) for permission. You will also need copyright permission to use images downloaded from the web, unless they are specifically labelled as copyright-free. There may be a fee for the use of copyright material.

16

Tips for bar charts, pie charts, flow charts and line drawings

Bar charts, histograms, pie charts, flow charts and line drawings are appropriate for many types of data and can help to make your poster more interesting.

Use bar charts where the independent variable is discontinuous . . .

Use bar charts where the independent variable (the X axis) is a category rather than a measurement (i.e. is discontinuous). For example, you might be comparing the effects of two different treatments on a single outcome in three different groups. Treatment effect (the continuous dependent variable) would be measured on the Y axis, so there would be three sets of paired bars.

. . . But do not use bar charts for logarithmic data

Logarithmic axes on bar charts do not make sense, as the point of a bar chart is to compare the height of the bars. Find a different way to represent logarithmic data.

Histograms have two measurable axes

Strictly speaking, the term histogram is applied to bar charts that have two measurable axes. Often such data are better expressed as a line graph, but histograms may be better for data collected at uneven intervals, e.g. 1 day, 1 week, 1 month, 2 months, 6 months.

Very simple bar charts are acceptable if they help to add interest to the poster

In a paper, most journals would be reluctant to accept bar charts with just two or three bars – the editors think such illustrations take up too much space for the amount of data presented. On a poster, however, you are in control. Go ahead and use a simple bar chart if you think it will help the reader to understand your results and make your poster more attractive to look at.

Add selected p values as appropriate

If you are making statistical comparisons between bars, you can include p values on the bar chart, using lines to indicate which bars are compared. If there are several such comparisons, you may prefer to use asterisks to indicate p values. You can then explain them in a key close by (preferably on the graph itself rather than in the figure caption; *see* Chapter 15). The usual sequence is $^*p<0.05$; $^{**}p<0.01$; $^{***}p<0.001$.

Add error bars as appropriate

Error bars may be needed on some bar charts. Make it clear in the key or figure caption what they represent (e.g. standard error, standard deviation or confidence intervals).

Avoid patterns on bars if you can use colour instead . . .

Although Excel and PowerPoint have many patterns available, colour is usually a better way of distinguishing between bars. Remember that you can get some pleasing and tasteful effects by using tints of a colour (i.e. less than 100%) or adding a small percentage of black to make the colour darker. This might be appropriate, for example, if you are comparing different doses of the same drug or different concentrations of the same reagent.

. . . But don't forget that you may need A3 colour handouts

There is no point photocopying your poster in black and white if you have used colour as one of your main differentiating features.

Avoid 3-D bars unless you have 3-D data

3-D bar graphs may look attractive at first sight, but we would advise avoiding them – statisticians hate them, and they look odd if you try to add error bars to them. Normal 2-D bar charts are fine.

Horizontal bar charts can be helpful if the axis labels are too long to fit on the X axis . . .

For some data categories, you may have rather long axis labels. In this case, horizontal bars may work better – i.e. with the X axis vertical and the Y axis horizontal. This is perfectly permissible and avoids the problems with readability posed by vertical or sloping axis labels. For example, you could use a horizontal bar chart if you were giving numbers of patients with particular diagnoses and the names of the conditions were too long to fit comfortably on a horizontal X axis.

. . . But do not display the same type of data in two different formats

Do not use horizontal and vertical bar charts on the same poster just to add variety – it is confusing for the reader if the same type of data is displayed in two different ways.

Use negative bar charts for negative scales

If your data consist of negative values – for example, if you want to indicate a reduction in a particular variable – it helps the audience to understand the bar chart if you construct it with the X axis at the top instead of the bottom.

Remember that you can subdivide bars

If your categorical variable divides into subcategories, you can subdivide bars horizontally to show subgroups within a single group (for example, men and women). It often works well to use tints of a single colour to indicate the different groups.

If you subdivide bars, put the darkest colour at the bottom

In bars that are subdivided horizontally, the darkest tint should be at the bottom, or an optical illusion will make the bar look top-heavy.

Pie charts show subdivisions within a single dataset

Pie charts are useful for showing the proportions of subgroups within a single dataset. For example, you might have a main category of '*Hospital admissions 2008–9*', and this could be divided into subcategories by diagnosis or by age group.

Do not have too many slices in your pie

Pie charts become hard to understand when there are more than about seven slices. If you have too many subgroups, you could consider combining some of the smaller ones as 'other'. If you need to, you could then use a linked pie or 100% bar to expand subcategories within a single slice.

Do not use a 3-D pie chart

Although 3-D pie charts look pretty, it is difficult to see the actual proportions of the slices.

For emphasis, cut a slice or use colour

To emphasise a particular value, you can cut a slice out of the pie or use a strong colour.

Start your slices at 12 o'clock and put them in a logical order

It is usual to arrange your slices in a logical order, starting at the top of the chart (12 o'clock) and working clockwise. What constitutes a logical sequence depends on your data, but it should not be random – readers will assume that there is some reason why the slices are in a particular order.

It is usually better to label slices rather than use a key

A key requires too much effort from the audience, so try to label the different slices instead. Text labels are often too large to fit neatly inside all the slices of the pie, so put them on the outside, arranged next to the relevant slice.

Consider adding percentages to your slices

If you think some readers will be interested in exact values, you can add percentages. They can go next to the labels, or if the slices are big enough, they can go inside the slices, with the category labels on the outside.

Do not ask readers to compare multiple pie charts

You can put two or more pie charts side by side, but it is very difficult for the reader to compare from one to another. If you want to compare frequency data, consider using 100% bars.

Use 100% bars to show more than one dataset on the same graph

An easier-to-interpret and space-saving option is to use 100% bars (like a rectangular cake sliced horizontally). This allows you to compare several different datasets.

Use flow charts to show processes or hierarchies

Flow charts can show processes (e.g. steps in an experiment) or hierarchies (e.g. taxonomic divisions of living organisms). When reporting randomised controlled trials in medicine, it is common to include a flow chart to show the numbers of patients in different groups at different points in the study.

Simple line drawings can be used to make your study design clear

Where appropriate, simple line diagrams are a useful way of showing the design of a study. For example, you might want to show dose titration schedules or a crossover design for a randomised controlled trial.

You can combine photographic images with line drawings to illustrate processes, hypotheses or models

Some topics lend themselves to 'pictorial' flow charts – for example, the life cycle of a parasite.

Line drawings may sometimes be clearer than photos

Line drawings are often clearer than photos – for example, if you are trying to show an anatomical feature, the construction of a piece of equipment or a surgical procedure. However, they are more time-consuming to produce, so be selective about what you choose to illustrate.

Edit the text on all charts and drawings ruthlessly to eliminate unnecessary words

Try to minimise the numbers of words on charts and drawings – this will give the reader less work to do and makes it easier to fit all the information you need into the space available. Think constantly about whether you can reduce the number of characters in a figure label. For example, could you substitute an upwards arrow for the word 'increased'?

17

Tips for photos

Good-quality photos can add greatly to the impact of your poster. On the other hand, poor photos can confuse or irritate readers. So it is worth making a big effort to ensure that your photos communicate not only a clear scientific message but also a professional image for you and your institution.

Select your photos according to their priority and purpose
Photos are very appealing to readers, but you may need to strike a balance between 'need to have' and 'nice to have'.

Your top priority should be photos that add to the science . . .
Some photos may illustrate your main results – for example, a gel or radiograph. These are your most important photos and you need to allow plenty of space for them.

. . . Or provide other scientifically relevant information
Other photos may be helpful but not strictly essential – for example, a photo of your experimental set-up, the organism you work on, or a clinical picture to illustrate a disease. These can add interest and make the study easier for readers to understand.

Your second priority should be photos that attract readers, rather than adding to the science

It is acceptable, within reason, to add photos purely to make your poster more visually interesting – for example, you could use a photo of the environment you worked in, your institution or the members of your team. Only include these if you have plenty of space and need an additional way of attracting readers' attention.

Use original images rather than scanned images wherever possible

For most scientific images, e.g. photos of gels or organisms, you will be working with images from a digital camera. Avoid scanning in images wherever possible, as the final printed, enlarged image may be unacceptably fuzzy.

If you must scan images, do so at high resolution

Photos should be scanned at 150 dpi at 100% of the final size they will appear on the poster. If you are working on a template that will need to be enlarged before printing, pictures should be scanned at 300 dpi. Images should be saved as high-quality .jpg files.

Be careful about sizing and colour intensity to allow comparisons

If you are asking readers to compare two sets of photographic data, e.g. gels, the photos must be placed on the poster so that they are at exactly the same relative scale and colour intensity.

Make sure you include a scale . . .

It is very difficult to interpret the relative size of objects on a photo. Make sure that you do not accidentally trim a scale from the corner of your photo. If no scale exists, make sure that you add one.

. . . And add appropriate labels

You may have looked at hundreds of gels or micrographs, so the features on the photos will be easy for you to spot. Someone reading your poster may not be as familiar with the content, so make sure that you superimpose clear labels on all major points of interest relevant to your study.

. . . But do not put too much writing over the image

If you need to label many features on your photo, consider putting small clear letters (A, B, C, etc.) on the photo itself and having a key to the lettering. This will avoid text and associated arrows obscuring the image.

Do not assume that what looks good on your monitor will print well

Poorer quality images may look fine on a computer screen but will look terrible on a full-size poster. If you are not sure how an image will look like when printed full size, click on it and then zoom in 200%. If it is fuzzy on your monitor, it will be fuzzy on your poster.

For the best-quality images, stick high-resolution prints onto your poster

We do not advise that you assemble the whole poster the old-fashioned way with bits and pieces stuck together. However, there are times when you may want a much higher resolution photo than the standard 300 dpi at which most posters are printed. In this case, print your photo at 1200 dpi on high-quality photographic paper and stick it carefully onto the poster.

Consider whether your photo needs a keyline around it

It often really improves the look of a photo to add a very thin black or grey border, especially if the photo itself has a light-coloured background.

Do not use photos of people without their permission

If someone can be identified from a photo, e.g. a patient, you should always have his or her written permission to use the image. It is not necessary, however, to obtain permission to use photos of isolated body parts.

Mask names on radiographs and other patient charts

If a patient's name appears on a radiograph, EEG, ECG or other clinical picture, you should mask it – again, it is part of your duty of patient confidentiality.

Do not use photos for which you do not have copyright unless you have obtained permission

It is tempting to use photos found on the Internet or to scan in photos from books or papers (but see above for practical problems with doing this). However, remember that you should have the original owner's permission to use their images. The copyright to papers is often held by the journal publishers, so you should write to them for permission. They will almost certainly request that you also write as a courtesy to the author of the paper. You may have to pay a fee for the use of a copyrighted image.

Acknowledge photos obtained from other people

You may need to put an acknowledgement next to photos from other sources (do not forget you can put this in small type at the side of the photo if it would otherwise make your photo caption too long).

Do not forget to indicate points of interest with arrows or rings around key features

In contrast to a presentation, you might not be around in person to point to the most interesting area of your photo. So make sure that you label any key areas of interest with a ring or arrow to attract readers' attention.

Consider adding a photo to help identify the presenting author

At a busy poster session, when lots of people are milling around your poster, it can be hard for people to identify you as the presenting author. It can be helpful for you to include a little passport-style photo of yourself so people can spot you. (Large photos may make you look slightly self-obsessed!)

Be careful with photos used as background images

If you really think it is a good idea, you can use 'watermark' background pictures appropriate to your topic – for example, fish scales for fish research. This sometimes works, especially if your poster is otherwise visually boring. However, we have seen many otherwise excellent posters that were spoiled by 'background overkill'. It is all too easy for a background to impede the readability of text or to detract from important figures. If you have plenty of other visual material on your poster, do not use a photographic background as well.

If you have a lot of photos to show, consider displaying them with a digital photo frame . . .

Digital photo frames are now relatively inexpensive and give you the option to include one or more gigabytes of photos on a repeating cycle. They usually have a hook or loop on the back for attaching them to the wall. You could adapt this to attach the photo frame to your poster, or you could simply use double-sided sticky patches. You will probably want to make the digital photo frame more secure with a motion alarm and/or security cable, as used for laptops.

. . . Or even on your laptop or mobile phone

A laptop gives you the chance to display not only photos but also video or animations, which are highly relevant for some sorts of data. Do not leave your laptop running and walk away, but when you are going to be there to watch over it, it could give an extra dimension to your poster. It is best to attach your laptop to a nearby heavy object (such as the poster stand) with a security cable – you can get security cables that include a motion alarm that makes a loud noise if anyone tries to move the laptop. Practise first to make sure you are not likely to set off the alarm yourself by accident and annoy everyone. Another possibility during the periods when you are standing by your poster is to have some extra images on your mobile phone to show people.

18

Editing and proofreading your poster

Once you have written your poster, it is a good idea to put it away for a couple of days and then to look at it afresh with an editorial eye. Use the checklist provided in Appendix 8 to help you. Your poster will require editing for its overall look, scientific content, spelling and grammar, flow of language and suitability of the design and layout for the data. If you have written the poster, it is very difficult to edit it yourself. Be prepared to let other people read and criticise your poster, and then address their comments in subsequent drafts.

Edit your text, figures and tables before importing them into PowerPoint

If you have written your text and tables in a word processing program, and your figures in another program, it is a good idea to edit them before you import them into PowerPoint. Once you are sure that your material is correct, you should only need to focus on layout once you have imported the text, figures and tables into PowerPoint.

Use automatic checking features in your word processing program . . .

Using the automatic spelling, grammar and readability checking features in your word processing program, before you import your main text into PowerPoint, will indicate obvious errors and areas that need attention.

. . . But you must also read the text

Spell-checkers in word processing packages will not pick up correctly spelled words used in incorrect contexts, such as 'their' and 'there' or 'forward' and 'foreword'. In addition, the computer programmers did not specifically program for scientific language and phraseology. The software may highlight some terms as incorrect when they are correct in your scientific context.

Check complex scientific terms carefully . . .

Look at long chemical names, strings of base pairs and scientific equations. Sometimes word processing packages have problems managing these.

. . . And familiar words even more carefully

It is easy to miss incorrect spellings in words that you know well. Look particularly at names of drugs, organisms, genes etc. Check all abbreviations and acronyms (CSF can easily become CFS).

Consider whether you are happy with readability and flow

Do you like what you read? Has your poster told the story that you want it to tell?

Choose two reviewers . . .

In addition to reading the manuscript yourself, it is a good idea to ask at least two other people to read it, because you will not spot your own inconsistencies and errors. You need people with differing skills.

- Choose *a colleague with good language skills and an eye for detail*. This person should read the manuscript for flow, readability, language, spelling, grammar, style and effectiveness in getting the message across.
- Choose *a senior scientist who has a good understanding of your data*. This person should read the manuscript for whether you have met your stated objectives, the validity of your conclusions and the scientific accuracy of your data. He or she should specifically look for data errors or omissions and should be asked to assess whether you have chosen the right way to represent your data.

. . . And tell each reviewer what is expected of him or her

You do not want the senior scientist spending time correcting spelling when what you need is input on the interpretation of the data.

Wait until you have both sets of comments before making changes to your poster

There will be occasions when the reviewers disagree, and you will need to balance the importance of their comments before making changes.

Read reviewers' comments with humility

If the reviewers appear to be confused by your poster, do not assume they are stupid! You have probably not conveyed your ideas in a way that makes it easy for the reader.

Redraft and reread your poster manuscript before importing it into PowerPoint

Make sure that you are completely happy with the scientific content and editorial accuracy of the poster before you transfer it into PowerPoint. It is much easier to make editorial changes in a word processing package than in PowerPoint.

In PowerPoint, proofread the layout

Once the poster has been designed in PowerPoint, print it out in colour on A3 paper. You should then do the tedious but essential job of proofreading.

Do a word-for-word check . . .

If you have written your poster in a word processing package, check that every word and symbol has transferred correctly into PowerPoint. Try to look only at the words, not letting your mind flow forward by reading the sentences. Some proofreaders do this by reading backwards from the end of the manuscript, which helps them to focus on individual words rather than on content. This should identify any 'cut and paste' errors.

. . . Then do a slow and careful read through for content and style

This time read your poster layout from beginning to end, imagining that you are seeing it for the first time.

Read titles, headings and captions carefully

It is difficult to spot errors in titles, headings and captions until the poster is printed full size, and then they are very obvious! Pay particular attention to any text in CAPITAL LETTERS. Read each title and heading as if you were seeing it for the first time.

Check for formatting errors

In the transfer from one electronic format to another, formatting errors can creep in. Check that:

- fonts are consistent and correct
- word, line and paragraph spacing is consistent
- text is left-aligned
- bold, italic and underlining commands have transferred correctly
- special symbols, e.g. $\geq$, $\leq$, $\pm$, $\circledR$, have not been lost
- superscripts and subscripts are correctly formatted.

Look carefully at graphs and charts

Check that:

- all the data points are present
- no information has become obscured or misaligned
- all the colours work effectively
- any keys are present and match the relevant graphs
- figures are associated with the correct captions
- figures are positioned (where possible) near to their related text
- footnotes are legible and adjacent to the correct figure.

Scrutinise tables

Look very carefully at the tables to ensure that:

- all the rows and columns have their correct headings
- data points are in the correct columns and rows
- everything is correctly aligned
- superscript and subscript numbers and symbols are correctly formatted
- tables are associated with the correct captions
- tables are positioned (where possible) near related text
- footnotes are legible and adjacent to the correct table.

Check photos

If you have used any photos, you must check whether:

- the resolution is appropriate
- they are sized and cropped correctly
- the labels are legible and superimposed correctly
- the scale bars on micrographs can be read
- the enlargement used is indicated.

Check references

If you have included any references on your poster, read slowly through each reference looking for errors in formatting. Check that if you used bold or italic for journal names, these have transferred correctly. Then stand back and check that the references are an appropriate size that is readable but not dominating.

Think about colour

Do you like the colours that you have chosen? Look at the colours of headings, text boxes, lines on graphs and bars on bar charts. Does your use of colour help or hinder the readability and flow of the poster?

Assess the overall layout

Do you like it? If you have used additional graphics, such as arrows between sections, do they help or hinder flow? Do you find it easy to find your way around the poster?

Check any additional audiovisual material

If you are adding an audio device or using a laptop as part of your presentation, check that it works and that the program runs effectively. If you are attaching a device to your poster, have you left space for it? Check the device several times in rapid succession to mimic delegates pressing the button.

Repeat the review process, this time on the PowerPoint layout . . .

Do not expect your reviewers to squint at a tiny A4 printout of a large poster layout. Give each of them an A3 colour version of the poster to read. If possible, give them copies of any additional audiovisual files so that they can get a feel for the entire poster.

. . . Again select a colleague with an eye for detail

This person should read the entire poster slowly and carefully from start to finish and consider whether it still makes sense. They should look for readability; effectiveness of the layout; flow of the story; format, size and impact of figures, tables, diagrams and photos; utility of any audiovisual material; use of colour and language; and spelling and grammatical errors.

. . . And a senior scientist

This person should do a critical read for scientific accuracy and should assess whether the layout and any additional audiovisual material add to or detract from the message of the poster.

Incorporate reviewer comments

Incorporate all the reviewer comments that you agree with. Do not rush any changes made at this stage – you do not want to add any additional errors. Carefully check your own work.

Check that changes made in response to comments have not affected your layout

If you have added or deleted text, it may have affected the number of lines in a text box, causing your layout to become unbalanced or text to overlap with other elements such as graphs. 'Widows' or 'orphans' (*see* Chapter 8) may have appeared. Often editing out just a word here or there can eliminate an unnecessary extra line of text and make everything fit nicely again.

Double-check that you have instructed PowerPoint to print at the correct size

If your page setup is incorrect, change it now. But remember that you will have to reread the entire poster, as the change in setting may have altered the layout.

Do a final read-through

You have to take responsibility for the poster, so you must undertake this final read. Print the final version in colour on A3 paper and read it slowly and carefully. Have you made all the corrections accurately? Are you happy for this version to go to print?

Save the final version and make it clear which electronic version is the one for print

Once you are happy that you have a final version of your poster, make sure that you could not inadvertently use an earlier version for printing. Create two folders on your computer: (1) Poster Archive and (2) Poster for Print. All previous versions of the poster should go into the archive. Only one file – the final print version – should be in Poster for Print. Put the date and the word 'final' into the file name of the print version.

Make a backup

You have done all this work, so it would be a shame to lose it now. Transfer the final print file onto a memory stick or CD and take it home, or back it up on the Internet. If your lab or office burns down, you can still go to the conference!

19

Printing your poster

You have reached the last hurdle – you have checked everything you can possibly check, you have saved the poster in the right format and you are ready to go. Here are a few tips to help you get your poster printed without problems.

Select a print supplier

Some institutions have in-house printers, but often you will need to find a local copy shop. It may also be possible to print the poster in the country of your conference if you are going overseas. This will save transportation but is risky, as you cannot check the quality before you go. Some conference organisers offer a poster production service (at a cost). If you accept this, be sure to follow their guidelines for submission of text, figures and tables.

Talk to your print supplier as soon as possible . . .

Try to avoid last-minute printing, as this can compromise the quality of the printed poster. As soon as you know when your poster will be ready, tell your print supplier. Ideally you should leave yourself enough time to reprint the poster if there are any print problems.

. . . Ensure that they can handle PowerPoint files

Most print suppliers who work directly with scientists will be able to work with PowerPoint files – though it is worth checking that your versions of PowerPoint are compatible. However, some print suppliers will be more used to receiving Quark files from design agencies. Check that the printer can handle the type of file that you have produced.

Double-check enlargement calculations

If your poster is not A0, you will have had to set the page size within PowerPoint to a fraction of the required final size, with a view to enlarging the poster at the print stage. Make sure that you tell the print supplier the exact enlargement that is needed – otherwise you will have a very small printed poster.

Specify landscape or portrait

Be clear about the format, as this will have a bearing on the paper stock available to you. Your print supplier may not look at your PowerPoint file before printing, and so would not immediately see your on-screen formatting.

Discuss the colours that you have used

Tell your print supplier if you have used a large amount of a strong or unusual colour on your poster. The printer may have to source additional inks. Very dark background colours can prove expensive to print and may require additional time to dry. Large areas of dark colour can also be patchy when dry, giving a poor-quality finish.

Choose good-quality paper . . .

Paper comes in different weights / thicknesses (measured in grams per square metre; gsm) and coatings. Each type of paper has different levels of absorbency for ink, so colours will seem slightly different on different papers. On poor-quality thin paper, ink is likely to run, and paper will curl when in contact with the wet ink. There is also a risk of the paper ripping when the poster is moved. Thinner paper is more transparent than thicker paper, reducing the contrast between the white paper and the printed text and reducing the perceived quality of the printed item. Print suppliers used to creating scientific posters will be able to advise you on the optimal type and weight of paper.

. . . And check that your chosen paper is available

Check that the print supplier has stocks of A0 paper in your chosen weight or can organise larger print sizes if required.

Consider the finish . . .

The finish of the poster can alter the overall look. You can choose matt or gloss finish. A gloss finish is often chosen to provide visual clarity.

. . . And think about lamination

Lamination entails covering the printed poster in thin plastic. It increases durability but costs more, adds time to the printing process and makes the poster more difficult to roll and transport. If you want a matt paper finish, do not bother with lamination. Consider lamination if you want to bring your poster home with you and use it again.

Leave enough time to reprint the poster if needed

Check the poster carefully before accepting it from the print supplier. There are occasions where the printed item is poor quality. If the paper is creased, torn or discoloured, or the fonts or colours are blurred, ask the printer to reprint it. Having worked so hard on the science, writing and editing, do not accept a poor-quality printed item.

Let the ink dry before transporting the poster

Do not be impatient. Ink needs time to dry completely, and dark or strong colours take longest. If you roll up your poster and put it in a tube or portfolio carrier before the ink is dry, there will be a very smudged and poor-quality poster at the conference.

Print A3 colour handouts of your poster

Be sure to specify colour copies, as the meaning of your data could be lost on black and white copies. You should only need a maximum of 25 handouts. If you run out when you are at the meeting, you can pay to have a few more copies made in the conference business centre or through your hotel.

Check the costs of producing handouts

Check the cost of producing handouts with the printer supplier, as it might be surprisingly expensive. For small numbers of handouts (e.g. 25), it might be cheapest simply to print one A3 colour copy on your laboratory printer and then make A3 colour photocopies.

Check the opening times of your print supplier

Be sure that you are able to pick up your poster and handouts when you need them. Think carefully about using overseas suppliers if you need to pick the poster up over a weekend or public holiday. You may find that the print suppliers are closed.

20

Transporting, displaying and presenting your poster

You have put a lot of work into creating a good poster, but having a printed poster in your hand is only part of the story. Next, you have to get it there. Most people take their poster and handouts with them to the conference, but you may be in a situation where your poster has to be couriered to you. And once you get to the conference, do not simply abandon your poster in the poster hall. You have worked hard to create it, so put in the time and effort to make the poster work for you.

A strong cardboard poster tube is ideal for transport . . .
Make sure you have a suitable means of transporting the finished poster. Do not fold your poster. If possible, roll it up and put it into a strong cardboard poster tube. These work well if you are going on any form of public transport, particularly on a flight. Poster tubes can usually be taken into an aeroplane cabin, but will survive in the hold if necessary.

. . . Though a portfolio carrier also works
Alternatively, you can keep your poster flat inside a portfolio case or even two large pieces of stiff cardboard taped together. This works if your poster is A0, though these options are not suitable for anything larger and are unwieldy on public transport. Portfolio carriers are not an option for aeroplane travel – they are likely to get damaged in the hold and are the wrong dimensions for hand baggage.

Clearly label your poster tube/portfolio carrier

If, for any reason, you become parted from your poster, you stand a chance of getting it back before the conference if you have labelled it with your name, the full postal address of your hotel *or* the full postal address of the congress centre, the title of your poster and the poster number. Mark portfolio carriers with 'Do not bend'.

Keep laptops and audio devices close to you when travelling

If you are adding an audio device or using a laptop as part of your poster presentation, package it carefully and keep it with you throughout the journey to the conference. Do not send these by courier.

Be able to track your courier package

You may need to have your poster sent to you at the conference by courier. If so, make sure that you have the telephone number of the courier and the consignment number of your parcel so that you can track its progress.

Take an electronic copy of your poster with you

If the main printed poster goes missing in transit, it is not a disaster. Most large congress centres have the capability to print posters or can recommend a local copy shop. If you have your poster on a CD or memory stick, it is relatively simple to get another printed version.

Take some means of fixing your poster to the board

Many conferences provide pins or sticky tape for attaching posters to the poster board. However, if you arrive late, you may find that all the fixing devices are used. Make sure that you find out what the poster board is made of and take appropriate fixing material with you. If you are travelling to the meeting, keep the fixings with your poster.

Use strong fixing materials . . .

You can fix your poster to a board using pins, double- or single-sided sticky tape, hook-and-loop tape or pressure-sensitive adhesive. Make sure that you take plenty of the strongest of these available. Unfortunately, posters that have been carried in poster tubes tend to curl and pull themselves away from their fixings. Make sure you take sufficient fixings to hold your poster flat against the board.

. . . Particularly if you are attaching an audio/video device to your poster

Although most audio/video display units are small and light, they need to be attached securely, particularly if the delegates are to be allowed to press a button to see your results. Make sure you have thought through how you will fix such devices.

Do not attempt to balance a laptop on your knee

If you are using a laptop to augment the data on the paper poster, try to book a small table from the conference organisers rather than balancing the laptop on your knee or putting it on the floor.

Remember to take/charge batteries for electronic devices

It is unlikely that there will be a power supply close to your poster. Make sure that you have fully charged batteries available for all equipment. If you are going abroad, check that you have a charger and a power adapter for that country. You may need a transformer if your equipment is 240 volts and the local electricity supply is 110 volts.

Do not leave any audio/video devices or laptops on or near your poster overnight

These can disappear without trace. Ensure that any mounting device can be removed and replaced easily. Even during the day, you should secure devices with appropriate security cables or stay with them at all times.

Ensure your poster is neatly aligned on the poster board

It is most pleasing for readers if your poster is central on the poster board and is straight rather than crooked. Consider taking a measuring tape to help you to position the poster centrally on the board. If you have a large poster, get a colleague to help you – it can be tricky to handle.

Have colour A3 handouts available

You should aim to have A3 handouts of your poster available next to it. Try not to clutter up the area around the poster board with piles of paper. Most conference organisers can provide handout holders that hang off the poster board. If these are not available, take boxes or holders with you so that the handouts remain stacked neatly.

Consider handing out reprints of your papers

It is a good idea to have reprints of your papers (if they are on a similar subject to your poster) available at the meeting. This will allow you to provide additional information for interested delegates and increases your chances of getting your papers cited.

Ensure you are familiar with the content of your poster!

Before you go to the congress, make sure that you are completely familiar with the content of your poster and that you can explain it to one of your colleagues without stumbling over your words. This will allow you to present your poster to interested delegates without faltering or referring to notes or (even worse) reading your own poster in front of the delegates.

Try to stand by your poster during all breaks in the main sessions

This is particularly important if you are keen to meet potential collaborators or employers, or if you have a controversial poster that merits a lot of explaining and debating. If you have to leave the poster unmanned during busy periods in the poster hall, leave a notice pinned to the poster board to tell people when you will be back or where you can be found.

Stand slightly to the side of your poster

This makes it easy for delegates to read uninterrupted. You are not transparent!

Dress smartly . . .

You do not need to treat a poster presentation as a formal occasion, but do not be too casual. If you look smart, it implies that you are taking your data seriously. Remember that you may want a job from one of the people that you meet at your poster.

. . . And do not wear clothes that clash with your poster

While it would certainly be overkill to coordinate your clothes with your poster colours, it may improve your poster presentation if you wear clothes that are restrained in colour and do not clash badly with the colours of your poster.

Wear your name badge

This helps delegates to know whom to approach if they have questions.

Make eye contact and acknowledge those who approach your poster

Smile, but do not try to start a conversation unless the delegate approaches you (or unless you know him or her!). Shy people and those with only a passing interest in your data will move on if they feel that you are too keen to talk to them.

Wait until a delegate finishes reading before starting a conversation

If someone stands for several minutes at your poster, you can take it that they are interested and it is worth asking their opinion on the data.

Check whether there are specific poster presentation times . . .

As a poster presenter, you may be requested by the conference scientific committee to stand by your poster at specific times during the conference. Sometimes this is simply so that delegates know when to find you, and sometimes you are asked to give a short presentation. Every conference is different, so check the guidelines.

. . . And stand by your poster at the right time

Make sure you arrive well before the time slot, as the audience may arrive early.

If you have been asked to give a presentation of your poster, prepare it before you arrive at the conference

Unless you are very confident at presenting in public, plan and rehearse what you are going to say in the same way as for any other presentation. Do not assume that because it is 'only' a poster, it is not important – you need to make an assured impression. Make sure you have prepared answers to the most likely questions. If you have been asked to present in a formal 'Best of' poster presentation session, check whether you need to develop any PowerPoint slides.

Speak to the audience, not to your poster

Rehearse your presentation so that you can face the audience while speaking. This will make it easy for delegates to hear you, and it allows you to see whether you are losing your audience. Do not turn your back on the audience and face your poster while giving your talk.

Do not go into too much detail in your presentation

The written poster is available for anyone who wants the detail. Highlight the objectives, the main results and the conclusions in your talk. You do not need to go into details of methods (unless your poster is concerned with the development of a new method).

Take questions at the end of your presentation

Taking questions at the end of your presentation, rather than during it, helps you to maintain the flow of your presentation and ensures that only delegates with a special interest have to stay to listen to detailed questions.

Attend the poster prize-giving

Some congresses award prizes for the best poster. You should definitely attend the prize-giving if you have won a prize. It is courteous to the organisers. Also try to attend the ceremony even if you have not won. You can pick up tips on how to write a better poster.

When you get home, make the poster work just a little bit harder . . .

After the meeting, do not just heave a sigh of relief and put your poster in the bin or with all the others in a pile beside your desk. Consider how you can make the most of your poster. You may be the only person in your institution who has attended the conference. Why not tell your colleagues about it?

. . . Display the printed poster in your department

If you can find wall space, simply hang the poster in a prominent position for a few weeks.

. . . Email poster copies to friends and colleagues

Do not be embarrassed. Most will be interested, even if it is only to steal your design ideas.

. . . Use your institution's intranet

If your institution has an intranet, find out how to upload information and put an e-copy of your poster on the relevant page.

. . . Place your poster in your institution archives

Many institutions now have archives of publications, which can be accessed by internet search engines. If possible, place an electronic copy of your poster there. Ask your librarian how to do this. But check regarding 'prior publication' issues if the data have yet to be accepted by a journal for publication as a full paper (also *see* below).

. . . Think about the Internet

Consider making your poster available on the Internet if you feel that your data are important (and your co-authors agree). There may be a website managed by your institution, but alternatively you can create your own web page or put your poster up alongside a blog. New e-poster 'journals' are also springing up where you can place your poster online. However, be careful if some of the poster content has been submitted to a journal for publication – making your poster freely available before publication of the full paper could be construed as 'prior publication'. If in doubt, check with the journal to which you are submitting the full paper.

. . . Write for your institution's newsletter

Newsletter editors are usually desperate for copy. Volunteer to write a report of the conference that you have just attended, in which you can discuss the data in your poster and how it was received. If you have won a prize with your poster, you may find that you are front-page news. If it is an electronic newsletter, include a link to an electronic copy of your poster.

. . . And give as many talks as possible

People who organise journal clubs and other similar events are often looking for speakers. Why not volunteer to talk about your poster? After all, you have had an entire conference to rehearse your presentation! Do not forget to give away A3 handouts and to tell people how to access an electronic copy.

Save the template and use it again

If you have had good feedback on the layout of your poster, stick to a winning formula.

21

E-posters: the future?

Electronic poster presentations (e-posters) are now part of the established scientific programme of some major conferences. E-posters are web-page documents submitted and designed online by the authors. They include text, figures and images just as in traditional paper posters, and they can also include new media, such as videos – which makes them a flexible option for some types of research. E-poster sessions allow a large volume of information to be presented at a conference (in some cases, several thousand posters are presented electronically).

An e-poster is not a second-class poster . . .

Being selected for an e-poster presentation is not a comment on the quality of your work.

In fact, being offered an e-poster can be a good option, as there are fewer restrictions on word count and size of figures and tables. They are also easy for delegates to access, as computer workstations at the venue make your poster available at any time during the conference, not just during allocated sessions. There is the potential for e-posters to remain accessible online after the meeting, which could result in e-posters becoming citeable publications (though check regarding prior publication issues if the material has been submitted to a journal for publication).

. . . And can still generate interaction with colleagues

Having an e-poster does not mean that you lose the interaction with colleagues that traditional posters allow. Delegates can interact with authors via email or through online chat forums. In some cases, the chat forums are made available for several weeks after the conference. Most conferences hold face-to-face discussion sessions based on e-posters. Email contact between author and delegate also opens up the option of booking an appointment to discuss the data in more detail, perhaps in a more social setting than the main hall of a conference centre.

Check how your e-poster is going to be used

Often e-posters are just viewed by delegates online (sometimes at a special e-posters booth), but at some meetings they are projected and the presenter has the chance to talk delegates through them.

Draft your e-poster in a word processing package, not PowerPoint

Do not go to the trouble of creating a layout of your poster in PowerPoint. The poster design will be dictated by the poster-design software used by the conference. It is best to draft your poster in a word processing package and to prepare good quality image files of figures. These can all be 'cut and pasted' into the online poster design software. Alternatively, you can write your poster directly into the online system, but often there is no opportunity to print it out for review and proofreading.

Use the manuscript version of your poster for the review and editing stages

Make sure all the editing and review stages of poster production are carried out on the manuscript version. Do not upload your poster onto the online system until you have a version of your poster that you are completely happy with. It is much harder to review your poster online and then to make changes to the poster once it is on the system.

Follow the online conference guidelines for e-poster development

Each type of e-poster design software is different. Some allow a lot of flexibility in design and content, and others are quite restrictive. Unlike many word processing packages, e-poster data management systems are not necessarily intuitive to use, and although guidelines are provided, some are easier to follow than others. Make sure that you know exactly what you need to do before you start.

Check the submission deadline

Every conference is different. Some allow submission of an e-poster right up until the week of the conference, and others close submission a week or so beforehand. Make sure that you submit in plenty of time.

Do not wait for the submission deadline to create your e-poster

Like all online systems, e-poster data management systems slow down at times of high traffic. It can be very frustrating to create your e-poster on a slow system. Also, if you leave it until the deadline, there will not be enough time for proofreading and checking your uploaded e-poster.

Do not forget your username and password

Online data management systems require a username and password. Do not forget these – write them down somewhere safe. Once forgotten it is not always possible to retrieve them from the system or from the conference organisers. You do not want to have to re-create your poster unnecessarily.

Upload your data online

Many systems have templates available for input of text, figures and tables. Most of these are set up to have the standard sections of title, authors, introduction, materials and methods, results and conclusions. However, it is usually possible to add new sections as required.

Save your data regularly

Most systems offer you the opportunity to save when you have completed each element of your poster. Make sure that you do this. If you log off or allow the system to time out before you have saved, all your work in that session could be lost.

Be meticulous when inputting information

If you have to type text or tables into the system, make sure that you do not rush. Reread every word, character and number carefully – it is easy to introduce typing errors during data entry.

Check for 'cut and paste' errors

It is best to 'cut and paste' your poster text from a finalised, fully reviewed and edited manuscript file. When you do this, however, it is easy to duplicate text by pasting it twice into the document or to omit text because you were distracted before you had pasted it into position. Check for these 'cut and paste' errors by ensuring that the first and last word of every sentence is present and that all the figure and table captions are in place. If you have uploaded a figure or table, check that you have placed each one in the correct place in the document, next to its caption.

Check all special symbols

Special symbols (e.g. $\geq$, $\leq$, $\pm$, $\circledR$) may not transfer between the word processing package and the e-poster data management system. Check that each one is correct. Most systems provide a menu of standard text and scientific symbols for you to use when writing or editing text online.

Check all text formatting

Formatting that you placed in your word-processed document may not transfer to the e-poster data management system. Check all superscripts, subscripts, bold text, italics etc. It will be possible to reinstate these if they have gone missing during the uploading of the text.

If a photo of you is needed, use a recent one

Some systems ask delegates to upload a photo of the poster presenter. This is not just decoration; it is so that you can be identified at the conference. Make sure that the photo is a good current likeness, not a more attractive shot from several years ago!

Decide how to upload your tables

Some systems ask you to type your tables into a pre-prepared format. However, it is often possible to upload tables as graphics files. To do this, you will need to create a .jpg of your table. Do not forget that if you need to amend the table, you will have to create a new graphics file and upload again.

Save your graphics files in the correct format

Guidance will be given on what types of graphics files will be acceptable and what resolution they should be. Make sure that you respect the guidelines, as incorrect file formats will not display correctly. Most systems will accept .jpg files.

Create high-quality graphics files

Most online systems allow delegates to enlarge the figures and tables onscreen, to make them easy to read. High-quality graphics files are best, as they produce better-quality enlargements.

Remember the rules for good poster design

Because e-posters have fewer restrictions on length, it is possible to have more text, figures and tables than normal. While this may be useful, it is easy to forget the rules for effective poster design given in this book (*see* Chapter 10 and the checklist in Appendix 8). Resist the temptation to write a mini-paper – try to use the number of words, figures and tables that you would in a standard printed poster.

Accept any restrictions on design

Because of the nature of data management systems, there is little scope for individual creativity in terms of design. Do not try to force the system beyond its limits – you are likely to lose data and to have an odd-looking poster on-screen.

Give yourself plenty of time to create your e-poster

For most people, creating an e-poster is a new experience, so do not rush. It can be time-consuming and frustrating to get the poster looking right, so allow at least 2 days for uploading your poster and then checking it on-screen.

Make sure that you know how to save your draft e-poster

It is unlikely that you will finalise your poster in one session. Be sure to save your draft version before logging off.

Do a word-for-word comparison of your word processing file and your online poster

This is very tedious, but to be sure that all your text is present and correct, it is essential.

Read the entire poster on-screen . . .

Check that the poster reads coherently and says what you want it to say. Does it look good on-screen? Does it flow well?

. . . And ask a colleague to read it too

Ask someone with an eye for detail to read the entire poster. They should look for use of language, typographic and grammatical errors, flow of information and accuracy of scientific content.

Test out all the electronic functions

Most systems allow delegates to read at different levels of magnification and to enlarge the figures and tables. Check that your poster works well at all magnifications and that the tables and figures are legible at all sizes. If you have included video and/ or audio files, make sure that these work correctly.

Do not press the submit button until you are completely happy with the content

Many systems do not permit editing of the poster once it has been submitted. Make sure that at least one other person has looked critically at the poster online before you submit it.

Check your email for an acknowledgement

Most data management systems automatically send an email to acknowledge online submission. This is usually instantaneous, so there will be an email waiting for you a few minutes later. If you do not receive an email within 24 hours of submission, log in to the online submission system. Normally you will be unable to access your poster if submission was successful. If the system simply failed to register your click of the submit button, then click it again. If the system says that you have submitted, but you still have not received an acknowledgement, contact the conference organisers.

Example of a structured abstract

Effect of hot and cold drinks on thesis-writing performance in final-year research students

Joe Java, Janice Teacosy and Levi Lacteous, Institute of Beverage Research, University of Somewhere, Wherever. Email: joejava@somewhere.org.

Background: Research students commonly work long hours writing up their theses, while consuming various hot and cold drinks. However, the effect of such drinks on their writing performance has not been objectively measured.

Objectives: We studied the effects of tea, black instant coffee, a high-caffeine drink (BlueSheep™), and hot milk on writing performance and wakefulness in final-year biochemistry research students.

Methods: 40 students (habitual water-drinkers) were randomly assigned to four equal groups. They consumed one 200 mL cup of each drink at half-hourly intervals from 21.00 to 01.30 (total dose 10 cups), unsupervised in their student accommodation, while writing the introduction to their theses. Consumption was verified by tea bags or cans discarded, weight of coffee granules or volume of milk used. Writing stopped at 02.00. Writing performance was assessed using MS Word readability scores. Statistical analysis used the Eyeball Test.

Results: On average, tea-drinkers wrote shorter sentences, shorter paragraphs, and more readable prose than the other groups. Writing performance was poorest on all measures in hot-milk drinkers (Table); in this group, 5/10 students (50%) fell asleep for up to 2 hours.

Drink (n=10 per group)	Mean sentences/ paragraph	Mean words/ sentence	Mean Flesch reading ease*	Mean Flesch-Kincaid grade level[†]
Tea	5.2	19.2	49.1	10.1
Black coffee	10.1	30.0	35.2	12.3
High-caffeine drink	15.0	35.1	40.0	15.1
Hot milk	20.1	69.9	5.6	20.0

*Score from 0 (unreadable) to 121 (every sentence a one-syllable word).

[†]Indicates the number of years of education required to understand the text.

Conclusions: Tea appears to be the most useful refreshment for research students. Black coffee and the high-caffeine drink were less beneficial than tea for writing performance in our study but may help to maintain wakefulness. Hot milk adversely affects writing performance and causes drowsiness.

Abstract checklist

1 Did the named authors make a specific contribution to the study?
2 Is the title explanatory and (if possible) declarative?
3 Is the background/objective no more than two sentences?
4 Does the background briefly establish context, if space allows?
5 Does the objective clearly state the main question you set out to answer?
6 Does the objective repeat or paraphrase the title? (Try to avoid this.)
7 Are all abbreviations defined on their first use?
8 Are acronyms used sensibly?
9 Is any jargon included that could confuse the reader?
10 Have you included key information on materials and methods (e.g. population, organisms, cells, genes or proteins studied; dosages of drugs or chemicals used; study design of clinical trials)?
11 Are the results presented in a logical order?
12 Have you given key numerical data with p values or confidence intervals, if relevant?
13 Does every result have a corresponding method and vice versa?
14 Is the table/figure (if included) clear and readable?
15 Do negative results use a lot of the available space? (If so, minimise them.)
16 Does the conclusion extract the one or two most important points and answer the question?
17 Is the conclusion supported by the results?
18 Are the methods and results described in the past tense and the background and conclusions in the present tense?
19 Have you stated the trial registration number and acknowledged the funding source (if required)?
20 Has an independent researcher reviewed the abstract?
21 Does the abstract give a good impression of an interesting, well-conducted, worthwhile study?
22 Have you slept on it before the final edit and submission?

Examples of style for poster headings, main text and figure and table captions

This is a good, clean and simple font for headings – it is Arial bold

You can use Arial font for subheadings as well as main headings

You can also use a serif font for headings – this is Times New Roman bold

This is a heading in sentence case – it is simple to read and to write

THIS HEADING IN CAPITALS IS MUCH MORE DIFFICULT TO READ

This Heading is in Title Case; Note that You Do Not Put Capital Letters on All Words – Avoid this Tricky Format

You can highlight your headings by putting them in a shaded or coloured box and using white text

Or you can use a light tint or colour in the background with black lettering

You might want to centre your text within a box with a coloured border

Leave two lines of space above your heading and one line of space below your heading

This is where the text would start or the figure or table would appear. Note that the font used for the main text here is Times New Roman to contrast with the heading, which is in Arial. This contrast works well, but it is also possible to use just one font on your poster for both headings and main text. More than two fonts looks too complicated. Whichever combination of fonts you choose, be consistent. This text is left justified (aligned at the left margin only). This is often the best option for poster text because left justification avoids problems with word spacing.

You can also use a sans-serif font like Arial for your main text, as in this paragraph. This paragraph is fully justified (aligned at left and right margins). Note that the spacing between words is uneven. When you enlarge this to poster size, the amounts of white space between words can make the text difficult to read. Sometimes it appears that there are 'rivers' of white running through your paragraph.

Leave one line space after each paragraph. Do not put the paragraphs close together and then indent the second one. On a poster, this would result in large, visually unattractive blocks of text. In your main text, bullet points are often preferable to paragraphs.

You can also use bullet points under subheadings or within paragraphs

- This is a bullet point – it is a sentence or phrase highlighting your key point.
- Try to have no more than four bullet points in a list.
- If you need to make more points, then the absolute maximum is seven bullet points.
- Do not make the bullet itself large or fancy – though you could choose to make it coloured.
- Try to keep to one level of bullet points, as
  - Second level and . . .
    - . . . third level bullet points become confusing.

Figure 1. Figure and table captions should be in a different size or style of font so that readers can distinguish them easily from the main text. Italics work well, but could lead to problems if your figure titles have to contain Latin biological names or abbreviations for genes that are conventionally italicised. In that case you might prefer to use a contrasting font, e.g. Times New Roman if your main text is in Arial, or vice versa. Or you could use coloured text for your figure and table captions.

References should be in smaller type than the main text. Reference style is:

1. Bloggs J, et al. *J Miraculous Results* 2008; 1: 3–15.

Sample landscape PowerPoint poster template

Modified with permission from a poster template used by the Department of Biochemistry, University of Oxford. Downloadable from www.radcliffe-oxford.com/biomedicine.

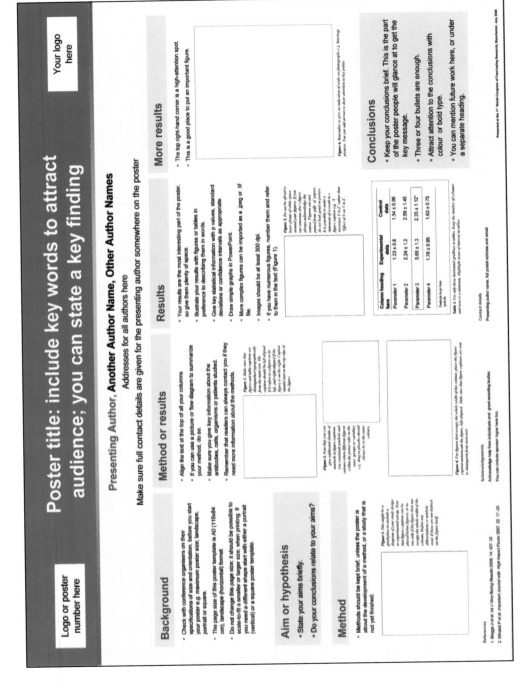

Sample portrait PowerPoint poster template

Modified with permission from a poster template used by the Department of Biochemistry, University of Oxford. Downloadable from <u>www.radcliffe-oxford.com/biomedicine</u>.

Poster title: include key words to attract audience; you can state a key finding

Presenting Author, Another Author Name, Other Author Names

Addresses for all authors here

Make sure full contact details are given for the presenting author somewhere on the poster

Background

- Check with conference organisers on their specifications of size and orientation, before you start your poster e.g. maximum poster size; landscape, portrait or square.
- The page size of this poster template is A0 (119x84 cm), landscape (horizontal) format.
- Do not change this page size; it should be possible to scale-to-fit a smaller or larger size, when printing. If you need a different shape start with either a portrait (vertical) or a square poster template.

Aim or hypothesis

- State your aims briefly.
- Do your conclusions relate to your aims?

Methods

- Methods should be kept brief, unless the poster is about the development of a method, or a study that is not yet finished.
- If you can use a picture or flow diagram to summarize your method, do so.
- Make sure you give key information about the antibodies, cells, organisms or patients studied.
- Remember that readers can always contact you if they need more information about the methods.
- Draw simple graphs in PowerPoint.
- More complex figures can be imported as a .jpeg or .tif file.
- Images should be at least 300 dpi.

Figure 1. This might be a good place to include a diagram of your study design or experimental set-up. Note that figure captions can be placed below figures, or to one side if the figure does not occupy the whole width of the column. Define any abbreviations or symbols used, if there are not defined on the figure itself.

References

1 Bloggs J et al. Int J Very Boring Results 2006; 14: 427–32.

2 Whotsit P et al. Important Journal with High Impact Factor 2007; 22: 17–25.

Results

- Align the text at the top of all your columns
- Your results are the most interesting part of the poster, so give them plenty of space.
- Illustrate your results with figures or tables in preference to describing them in words.
- Give key statistical information with p values, standard deviations or confidence intervals as appropriate.
- If you have numerous figures, number them and refer to them in the text (Figure 1).

Figure 2. Make sure that figure and table captions are distinguished typographically from the main text. The caption should be left aligned if it refers to a figure on its left, and right-aligned if the figure is on the right. Caption should start at the top edge of the figure.

Figure 3. Note that you can give additional details of methods in figure captions. Use consistent symbols and colours when different figures within the poster refer to the same groups or variables e.g. drug vs placebo should always be in the same colours.

Figure 4. For figures that occupy the whole width of the column, place the figure caption underneath the figure, left-aligned. Make sure that figure captions are easy to distinguish from main text.

Column heading here	Experimental data	Control data
Parameter 1	1.23 ± 0.8	1.34 ± 0.98
Parameter 2	2.24 ± 1.2	2.90 ± 1.46
Parameter 3	3.65 ± 1.3	2.36 ± 1.12*
Parameter 4	1.76 ± 0.96	1.63 ± 0.75

Footnote to go here
*p<0.05

Table 1. Use only basic horizontal gridlines in tables. Keep the number of columns and rows to a minimum. Highlight areas of interest in tables.

Acknowledgements

Acknowledge help from individuals and grant-awarding bodies.

You can include sponsor logos here too.

More results

- The top right-hand corner is a high-attention spot.
- This is a good place to put an important figure.

Figure 5. Do not be afraid to leave plenty of white space around your figures. If you use someone else's figure, always acknowledge the source. Figures cut and pasted from .pdfs of papers do not look good on posters. It is possible to make a statement of a result in a figure caption e.g. 'X increases Y in Z' rather than 'Effect of X on Y in Z'.

Figure 6. Remember to give an indication of scale in photographs e.g. histology pictures. You can add arrows to draw attention to key points.

Conclusions

- Keep your conclusions brief. This is the part of the poster people will glance at to get the key message.
- Three or four bullets are enough.
- Attract attention to the conclusions with colour or bold type.
- You can mention future work here, or under a separate heading.

Contact details

Presenting author name, full postal address and email

Presented at the 1st World Congress of Fascinating Research, Manchester, July 2009

Example of a creatively designed landscape poster

Note the restrained colour scheme and imaginative use of columns. The results and conclusions stand out strongly. Reproduced with permission of the authors and Scienceposters, www.scienceposters.co.uk.

Cytokine release from alveolar epithelial cells: a role for thioredoxin?

Imperial College London

SK Leaver, L Pinhu, M Griffiths, G Quinlan, TW Evans, A Burke-Gaffney

Unit of Critical Care, National Heart and Lung Institute, Faculty of Medicine, Imperial College London, London, UK

Royal Brompton and Harefield NHS Trust

Introduction

- Excessive cytokine production and perturbation of intracellular redox (reduction-oxidation) state contributes to the development of lung inflammation[1,2].
- Thioredoxin (Trx) is a ubiquitous thiol [sulfhydryl (-SH)] protein that regulates redox balance within cells[3].
- Trx is oxidised when it transfers reducing equivalents to disulphide groups in target proteins and it is reduced back to the dithiol form by an NADPH-dependent flavoprotein, thioredoxin reductase (Figure 1)

Figure 1: The thioredoxin system

NADPH   Trx-(SH)₂   Trx-(S)₂   Disulphide group of target protein [-S-S-]

NADP   TrxR-(SH)₂   TrxR-(S)₂   Dithiol (-SH)₂

Aims

- Thioredoxin expression is increased in pulmonary conditions associated with inflammation such as acute lung injury (ALI) and sarcoidosis[3,4].
- Previous studies have suggested that Trx might regulate cytokine release from cell lines including Mono mac6 cells (a human monocyte cell line) and endothelial cells[5].
- PMX464 (formally AW464) inhibits Trx cycling by forming an irreversible complex with the active site thiol groups in the reduced form of Trx.
- In this experiment we planned to investigate the role of Trx in cytokine release from Type II alveolar epithelial cells by inhibiting Trx pharmacologically using PMX464 and genetically using RNA interference.
- To investigate the role of Trx in cytokine release from A549 cells (a human type II alveolar epithelial cell line) using pharmacological and genetic methods of inhibition.

Methods

- A549 cells were treated with PMX464 (10µM) for 30 min. This was removed and then stimulated with IL-1β (1ng.ml⁻¹) for 24 h.
- Alternatively, A549 were transfected at 30-40% confluence (16-24h after seeding) using a mixture of Trx siRNAs from Dharmacon and Santa Cruz (20µM) with Genlantis Genesilence™ siRNA transfection reagent. Transfected cells were treated with IL-1 (3pg.ml⁻¹) for 24 h. Western blot analysis was used to confirm Trx knockdown was at least 70%. (Figure 2)
- Cell supernatants were analysed for IL-8 and GM-CSF concentrations, and for comparison levels of ICAM-1, by ELISA.

Results

- PMX464 reduced basal and IL-1β stimulated IL-8 (figure 3A) and GM-CSF release (Figure 3C). ICAM-1 expression was also significantly reduced following treatment with PMX464 (Figure 3B).
- By contrast, despite successful knockdown of Trx in A549 cells (Figure 2), expression of IL-8 in A549 cells (Figure 2), GM-CSF (Figure 3A), GM-CSF (Figure 3B) and ICAM-1 (Figure 3C) were not significantly reduced at baseline or following treatment with IL-1.

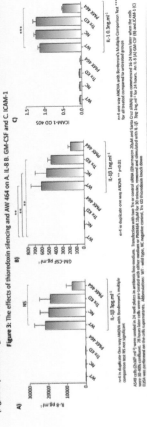

Figure 2: Thioredoxin knockdown in A549 cells.

Figure 3: The effects of thioredoxin silencing on AW 464 on A. IL-8 B. GM-CSF and C. ICAM-1

Conclusions

- PMX464 has potent anti-inflammatory properties in A549 lung epithelial cells, which were not reproduced by silencing thioredoxin expression
- This suggests PMX464 has other anti-inflammatory properties that might result from inhibition of other proteins with the thioredoxin motif in addition to thioredoxin OR that knockdown was insufficient to reduce thioredoxin activity enough to have an anti-inflammatory effect.

References

Acknowledgements

British Heart Foundation   wellcome trust

Example of a simple but effective portrait poster

Note that a one-column design like this only works if the text is large, so that there are not too many words per line. If you need to get more text on a portrait poster, at a smaller font size, it is better to use two or three columns (*see* Appendix 4). Reproduced with permission of the authors and Scienceposters, www.scienceposters.co.uk.

Incidence of post-discharge nausea and vomiting following day case gynaecological surgery

TL Gregory, S Jackson
Poole General Hospital, Poole, UK

Poole General Hospital **NHS**
NHS Foundation Trust

Introduction

- Up to 30% of day surgery patients may develop post-discharge nausea and vomiting (PDNV).
- Post-discharge opioid analgesia might contribute to the risk.
- We routinely discharge day surgery patients after laparoscopy with oral morphine but without anti-emetics.
- By contrast we discharge patients after hysteroscopy without opioids.
- We compared the incidence of PDNV in both groups.

Methods

- Data were collected from 50 consecutive patients by retrospective chart review and standardised telephone interview one week post-operatively.
- We calculated a risk score for each patient (0-4) using the simplified Apfel scoring system.

Results

- Seven of the 24 (29%) laparoscopy patients and six of the 26 (23%) hysteroscopy patients experienced PDNV (χ^2 ns).
- The duration of PDNV was greater in the laparoscopy patients (0-3 vs 0-1 days (χ^2 p < 0.05).
- Five of the 13 who took morphine had PDNV, three linked morphine to PDNV and one was readmitted due to PDNV.
- Two of the 11 who did not take morphine had PDNV (χ^2 ns).
- All patients who developed PDNV had received one anti-emetic before discharge and seven, two.
- There was no relationship between the incidence of PDNV and calculated risk score.

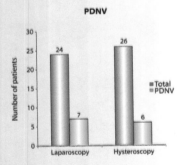

PDNV

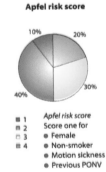

Apfel risk score

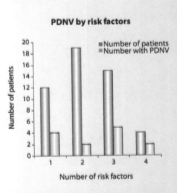

PDNV by risk factors

Conclusions

- An important number of our patients undergoing day case gynaecological surgery suffer PDNV.
- This may last longer after laparoscopy and post-discharge oral morphine.
- We have changed our policy on the basis of this study and will discharge these patients with ondansetron.
- The frequency and duration of PDNV will be re-examined later this year.